The Superhuman Lifestyle

A Guide to Mahn and Society in Sexual Crisis

Radheshyam More

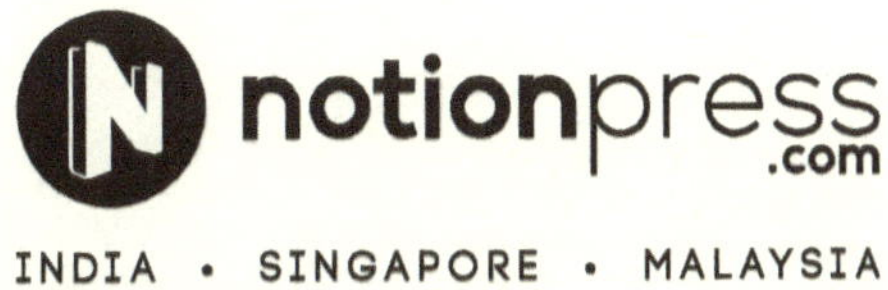

Contents

Preface

Join me on an incredible journey with this book, a treasure for everyone, regardless of age, background, beliefs, or job. It's like a bridge connecting us to wisdom from the past and hope for the future. The wisdom of great spiritual masters, who attained it through spiritual discipline, hard work, and sacrifices, should guide our lives. To pass on these values, we need to live by the teachings of our elders.

Creating a fulfilling life with discipline, health, joy, ambition, and purpose isn't just a good idea; it's crucial. If we don't, life can become filled with pain, worry, stress, and other challenges. This book explores an ancient concept called Brahmacharya, a lifestyle from wise sages of ancient India found in texts like the Vedas, Upanishads, Bhagavad Gita, Mahabharata, and more.

I wrote this book because I read a life-changing book called *"Divine Inspiration: The Secret of Eternal Youth."* It taught me about Brahmacharya, inspiring positive changes in my life. Eager to share this wisdom globally, I researched celibacy and how it can improve lives. This book emphasizes the importance of understanding and adopting the Brahmacharya Lifestyle in today's world, which we've named the **Superhuman Lifestyle** because it can transform your life from normal to superhuman.

The motivation behind this book is clear—to show the serious condition of today's generation, which indulges in premarital sex while ignoring Brahmacharya. Based on research and stories from millions of young people, the book highlights the harms of unhealthy habits like masturbation, porn addiction, and premarital sex. The lack of Brahmacharya education in schools contributes to this, as explicit content floods our lives through literature, movies, ads, and online platforms, especially on smartphones.

Smartphones, now a big part of young people's lives, contribute to unhealthy habits, disrupting organized living, time management, clear thinking, and learning from older generations. By disconnected from true guidance from great spiritual masters, young people often prioritize temporary pleasures, neglecting crucial aspects of life.

To address this, our society must teach Brahmacharya to children starting at 12. While adding it to school lessons poses challenges due to outside influences, individual education is still possible.

This book aims to make the concept of Brahmacharya clear, offering insights into its different aspects and how it applies to daily life. Following Brahmacharya promises a healthy, productive, and purposeful life for the next generation. I extend my gratitude to my team and the contributions of over one million ManthanHub followers, whose experiences have made this book practical, scientific, and phenomenal. May this book reach every young person, parent, teacher, and professional, guiding them toward a brighter future.

Best Regards,
Radheshyam More

CHAPTER I

The Cycle of Chasing Pleasure

Why do we enjoy the things we do? Why do we feel happy, sad, angry, or afraid? These are some of the questions that have fascinated philosophers, psychologists, and neuroscientists for centuries. But to fully understand the nature of our emotions and desires, we need to look beyond our brains and bodies and explore how pleasure can be enriching yet detrimental.

Pleasure is one of the most fundamental aspects of the human experience. It motivates us to seek food, sex, social bonds, art, music, and many other forms of gratification. But where does pleasure come from? How does it shape our emotions, preferences, and behaviors?

One of the main scientific reasons is that pleasure is hardwired into our brains. Pleasure activates our brain's reward system, which releases dopamine, a neurotransmitter that makes us feel good and motivates us to repeat the behavior that triggered it. Dopamine is essential for learning, memory, and survival, but it can also create a feedback loop that reinforces our cravings and habits. Dopamine also influences our emotions, attention, and decision-making, making us more impulsive and less rational when we seek pleasure.

In this book, I will show you how pleasure evolved as a way of motivating organisms to survive and reproduce, and how it influenced their behavior, cognition, and culture. I will also reveal how pleasure is not a fixed or universal phenomenon, but rather a dynamic and context-dependent one, that depends on our genes, environment, and social interactions. We will also look at how pleasure interacts with other aspects of our minds, such as cognition, memory, learning, and decision-making. Finally, we will consider how pleasure influences our social and cultural lives, as well as our health and well-being.

By understanding the evolution of pleasure, we can gain a deeper appreciation of its role in our lives and its implications for our future. We can also learn to enjoy pleasure more wisely and responsibly, without falling prey to its potential pitfalls and dangers.

So how can we break free from the trap of pleasure? One way is to cultivate a different kind of happiness is Eudaimonia which is a Greek word that means "human flourishing" or "living well". Eudaimonia is not based on pleasure but on meaning, purpose, virtue, and growth. Eudaimonia is achieved by living according to our true nature and potential, expressing our talents and passions, contributing to something greater than ourselves, developing our character and wisdom, cultivating positive relationships and emotions, and finding joy in the journey rather than the destination.

By the end of this book, you will have a deeper and richer understanding of yourself and others, as well as a new appreciation for life's diversity and beauty. You will also learn how to harness the power of pleasure to improve your health, happiness, and relationships. And you will realize that pleasure is not a sin or a vice, but a gift from nature that we should celebrate and cherish.

What happens when pleasure becomes a problem? When we lose control over our impulses and cravings, and end up harming ourselves or others? This is the dark side of pleasure, the realm of addiction and compulsion.

We will explore how addiction and compulsion hijack our brains, altering our neural circuits and chemistry in ways that make us more vulnerable to relapse and less able to resist temptation. We will also examine how different factors, such as genetics, environment, stress, and trauma, can influence our susceptibility to addictive and compulsive behaviors.

Finally, we will discuss some of the current treatments, lifestyles, and strategies that can help us overcome these challenges and restore our balance and well-being.

To illustrate these concepts, we will use some examples from real-life cases of people who struggled with addiction and compulsion. We will look at how the loss of vital energy through various evil practices has made millions of lives hellish. These examples will help us understand the common patterns and mechanisms that underlie different forms of addiction and compulsion, as well as the unique challenges and opportunities that each faces in their recovery process.

CHAPTER II

The Dark Side of Negative Pleasures

We have all have experienced negative pleasures at some point in our lives. These are the activities or behaviors that give us short-term gratification but have long-term negative consequences. For example, binge-watching a show, overeating junk food, procrastinating on a task, smoking a cigarette, drinking alcohol, gambling, porn addiction, masturbation addiction, and over-indulgence in sexual activities, etc. These negative pleasures may seem harmless or even enjoyable at the moment, but they can have serious repercussions on our health, happiness, productivity, relationships, and self-esteem.

Why do we engage in negative pleasures? There are many possible reasons, such as boredom, stress, anxiety, depression, loneliness, peer pressure, habit, addiction, or lack of self-control. Sometimes we may not even be aware of the negative consequences of our actions, or we may rationalize them away. We may think that we deserve a reward after a hard day, or that we can make up for our indulgence later. We may tell ourselves that it's not a big deal, or that everyone else is doing it.

However, these excuses do not change the reality of the situation. Negative pleasures have a cumulative effect on our well-being. They can impair our physical and mental health, lower our motivation and self-confidence, damage our relationships and reputation, reduce our opportunities and achievements, and increase our guilt and regret. They can also create a vicious cycle of dependence and dissatisfaction. The more we rely on negative pleasures to cope with our problems or emotions, the more we need them to feel good. The more we indulge in them, the less we enjoy them. The less we enjoy them, the more we seek them.

Some more examples of negative pleasure and practice include addiction, violence, self-harm, exploitation, pornification, promotion of sexual appeal, and sexualization of society. These behaviors can have detrimental effects on the individual, family, and society as a whole.

To illustrate how pleasure can be detrimental and manipulated to increase unrest in society, I would like to give one practical example of Dr. Miriam Grossman, who is a campus psychiatrist who has exposed the harmful consequences of political correctness in her profession in her book "Unprotected". She argues that campus health and counselling services are misleading students about the risks of sexually transmitted infections, abortion, and promiscuity, and neglecting to tell them the truth about the benefits of faith and family. We are giving here some of the shocking stats taken from her book *Unprotected*, such as:

- There are 15 million new cases of sexually transmitted infections every year in the U.S., and half of them occur among people aged 15 to 24.

- There are over a million abortions in the United States each year, and 52 percent are in women under twenty-five.

- A survey by the National Marriage Project revealed that 81% of young adults said that marriage was an important goal for them, but only 26% were married by age 30.

Dr. Grossman contends that campus counsellors and health providers should stop feeding students' platitudes about "safer sex" and "choice", and instead help them understand the physical, emotional, and spiritual consequences of their decisions. She also urges parents, educators, and policymakers to challenge the radical social agendas that have taken over campus culture and to promote a more balanced and realistic view of human sexuality and relationships[1].

I will be giving you various shivering experiences and the impact of various negative practices committed by my millions of students in the later chapters. The most crucial question is "How can we break free from negative pleasures?" The first step is to recognize and acknowledge them. We need to be honest with ourselves about what we are doing and why we are doing it. We need to identify the triggers and rewards that drive our behavior. We need to evaluate the costs and benefits of our choices. We must face the reality of the consequences of our actions.

The second step is to replace negative pleasures with positive ones. Positive pleasures are activities or behaviors that give us long-term satisfaction but have short-term challenges. For example, exercising, meditating, reading a book, learning a new skill, completing a project, helping someone in need of spiritual practice, etc. These positive pleasures may seem difficult or boring at the moment, but they can have lasting benefits for our health, happiness, productivity, relationships, and self-esteem.

We must acknowledge that positive pleasures have a cumulative effect on our well-being. They can enhance our physical and mental health, increase our motivation and self-confidence, improve our relationships and reputation, expand our opportunities and achievements, and decrease our guilt and regret. They can also create a virtuous cycle of independence and satisfaction. The less we depend on negative pleasures to cope with our problems or emotions, the less we need them to feel good.

How can we cultivate positive pleasures?

The third step is to plan and practice them. We need to be intentional and proactive about what we want to do and why we want to do it. We need to schedule time and space for our activities, and eliminate distractions and temptations. We need to monitor our progress and reward ourselves for our efforts. We need to seek support and feedback from others who share our interests or values. We need to embrace challenges and learn from failures. We need to celebrate successes and appreciate experiences.

In conclusion, negative pleasures are tempting but harmful, and positive pleasures are challenging but beneficial. We have the power and responsibility to choose between them. We can either succumb to short-term gratification or strive for long-term satisfaction. We can either live in regret or joy. The choice is ours. In the following chapters, you will learn about the practice that can immensely help you rewire your brain from negative habits to positive ones, which in turn develop superhuman qualities.

CHAPTER III

Endless Pleasure with the help of Brahmacharya

Brahmacharya is a Sanskrit term that means "conduct consistent with Brahman" or "on the path of Brahman". It is a practice of self-restraint and celibacy that aims to achieve physiological, psychological, and spiritual benefits and harmony. Brahmacharya has many positive effects on the individual, family, and society as a whole. Some of these effects are:

- It enhances one's physical, mental, and emotional health by conserving and channeling vital energy.

- It fosters a sense of detachment, purity, and devotion that helps one overcome futile worldly temptations and attachments.

- It strengthens one's moral character, self-discipline, and willpower, making one more capable of fulfilling one's duties and responsibilities.

- It cultivates a deeper connection with the divine, leading to higher wisdom, peace, and bliss.

- It promotes harmony, loyalty, and respect in the family, creating a supportive and nurturing environment for all members.

- It contributes to social welfare, justice, and harmony by reducing conflicts, violence, and exploitation caused by lust, greed, and selfishness.

I have done intense research on the concept of Scientific Brahmacharya and I can assert that Brahmacharya is one of the most powerful ways to transform your life and achieve lasting happiness. Brahmacharya is not just about celibacy or abstaining from sexual activity, but rather about cultivating a higher awareness of the true source of pleasure, which is within yourself.

Brahmacharya means living in harmony with Brahman, the supreme reality that pervades everything. It means aligning your thoughts, words, and actions with the highest truth and purpose of your existence. It means transcending the lower impulses of the mind and body that seek satisfaction in external objects and experiences, and instead finding joy and peace in your inner self.

Brahmacharya helps you reduce negative pleasures and increase the influence of positive pleasures in your life. By practising Brahmacharya, you can gradually withdraw your attention from the negative pleasures of the senses and focus it on the positive pleasure of the self. You can learn to discriminate between what is real and what is unreal, what is beneficial and what is harmful, what is essential and what is unnecessary. You can develop a sense of detachment and dispassion towards the harmful worldly attractions and distractions that keep you away from your true self. You can cultivate a higher taste for spiritual values and virtues that enrich your life and uplift your soul.

Brahmacharya is not a denial or suppression of pleasure, but rather a redirection and sublimation of it. It is not a rejection or avoidance of life, but rather a mastery and enhancement of it. It is not a sacrifice or renunciation of happiness, but rather a discovery and expression of it.

In the following chapters, I will share with you the basic science of Brahmacharya, the prerequisites of Brahmacharya, the importance of Brahmacharya as per modern Science & Ayurveda, and its uncounted practical benefits as well as some practical tips and techniques on how to practice Brahmacharya in your daily life. I will show you how to overcome the challenges and obstacles that may arise in your journey towards self-control and the practice of Brahmacharya. I will also share with you some inspiring stories and examples of people who have successfully practised Brahmacharya and attained the highest state of permanent & eternal pleasure in human life.

CHAPTER IV

The Blueprint for Achieving Peak Performance

Brahmacharya or celibacy is a logical way of saving and storing precious energy so that it can be used for other vital functions. And if it is saved like this, it can be transformed, just as solid, dense water is transformed into subtle steam. Then it can do amazing things. A river may not have much power on its own. You may be easily able to cross it by boat or by swimming. But, if it is blocked up and its waters stored, then it has the power, when properly directed, to spin large turbines and produce electricity. The bright sun, even in summer, does not usually cause a fire, but if you concentrate its rays through a lens, those rays will instantly burn whatever they are aimed at. That is what celibacy is. This is the reasoning behind celibacy.

If you save this vital energy and divert it to the spiritual process of thinking, studying and reflecting on philosophy, and meditating, it becomes successful, because you have focused your force, and you can direct the focused force by aiming it at your spiritual practices. If it is saved, focused, and diverted into a specific channel, it works wonders. I would cite an important conversation between a student and Swami Chidananda in the book *The Role of Celibacy in Spiritual Life.*

Question: Celibacy is often seen in the modern West as an outdated, old-fashioned practice. It is often seen as oppressive, life-rejecting— even contrary to what spiritual practice is ultimately about. Many spiritual experts in the West are now teaching that to realise our full potential as human beings, we must accept, rather than in any way avoid or suppress, our sexuality. These views stand in sharp contrast to what the great traditions have always taught. What do you think about this?

Swamiji said: I have a different perspective from the one that was just shared. I think they have not understood the role of Brahmacharya in the spiritual journey. It is not outdated; it is not old-fashioned, and it is not restrictive or negative. Rather, it is a tool for achieving eternal life, infinite life. Their vision of life seems to be very limited and narrow. There is more to life than this. When you get a glimpse or an idea of what real life is, you will be astonished. This current life is meaningless without the awareness of its purpose. It is a trivial thing, a nothing, if not seen as a preparation for that greater life.

This life is a means to that sublime, magnificent, noble goal and aim of human existence which is to attain a divine life that is in harmony with God's life, the Kingdom of Heaven. No one who has some religious knowledge and awareness or a spiritual outlook will ever reject the importance of Brahmacharya. It is something scientific and science never becomes obsolete or old-fashioned. Brahmacharya is neither avoiding sexuality nor repressing sexuality. It is transcending sexuality so that the potential and the power of the sexual process can now be used for something so amazing that sex becomes insignificant in comparison.

Brahmacharya does not mean suppressing or avoiding sexuality. It means channeling sexual energy for a higher purpose, something that can give us much more joy and fulfillment than sex. This is not a misunderstanding or a denial of our human nature. It is a recognition of our true nature, which is beyond human. We are not mere mortals; we are divine sparks. Our human existence is only a dim reflection of our real identity.

The only value of our human existence is that it can serve as a bridge to our divine destiny, and to the Kingdom that we belong to by right of birth. To illustrate the practice of celibacy in a way that is relevant to the modern mindset, think of an Olympic athlete who has a burning desire to win a gold medal. He will gladly follow the guidance of a coach, and if the coach says, "No more partying, no more sex, no more junk food, no more alcohol," the athlete will happily comply.

He says: "I'll do whatever you ask me to do." Why? Because he wants the gold medal. And nobody questions him, nobody criticizes him. Why? Because the gold medal justifies all these so-called "restrictions." You cannot say that he is harming himself or repressing himself, because he does not see it that way. He is willing to do anything that the coach requires of him. It is not forced upon him by others. We understand his motivation and we respect it.

The Western notion that Brahmacharya is a form of repression is not completely unfounded. Repressing or suppressing a natural impulse or faculty can have negative effects on one's personality. Forcing Brahmacharya on someone who does not want it or is not ready for it can create psychological problems, because the person is acting against their inner desire and will, either due to external pressure, social norms or premature vows that were not well thought out.

But if a rational person, after reflecting deeply on the purpose of life, decides: "I want to achieve something great, something sublime, and I cannot afford to waste the energies that I possess. The more I preserve, the more I can channel into that goal and the higher the probability of success." With this reasoning and understanding, and with a clear vision of the outcome, if they voluntarily, joyfully, and enthusiastically embrace celibacy, where is the question of repression?

Rather, what seems to be a restriction is a full expression of a higher dimension of your being that you have now entered. So, instead of denying self-expression, it is enhancing it, because you are no longer attached to the lower aspect of your total personality. You are aligned with the higher aspect. It is a kind of liberation and evolution to a higher level. It is something positive, creative, and not anything negative. It is not a denial but an actual expression of yourself in the form of a strong aspiration and a noble ambition.[2]

The pursuit of the Supreme Reality requires complete dedication and sacrifice of one's lower desires and attachments. This is the ancient and timeless path of Brahmacharya, which transcends the narrow and superficial views of Freud and others who could not imagine such a sublime goal. In this age of sensual indulgence and materialistic obsession, the practice of Brahmacharya is more relevant and urgent than ever. It is not only a moral virtue, but also a scientific method to harness the vital energy and channel it towards the realization of the Self. The benefits of Brahmacharya are manifold, both for the body and the mind, but the ultimate reward is the bliss of the spirit, which can only be attained by those who follow this noble way of life. Therefore, one should study and understand the science of Brahmacharya in depth, and not limit oneself to the superficial aspects of *Nofap (*not to fap*)*.

CHAPTER V

The Alchemy of Brahmacharya with Modern Chemistry

This chapter will examine the chemical composition and functions of seminal fluid, and how its preservation affects the health and happiness of the individual. We will also discuss the insights of Ayurveda, the traditional Indian system of medicine, on the role of seminal fluid in maintaining balance and harmony in the body and the soul.

According to RW Bernard's book *Science Discovers the Physiological Value of Continence*, semen is a rich and alkaline fluid that contains high amounts of calcium, phosphorus, lecithin, cholesterol, albumen, nucleoproteins, iron, and vitamin E. These substances are essential for the nourishment of the nervous and brain tissues. A normal ejaculation releases about 226 million sperm cells, which carry large amounts of lecithin, cholesterol, nucleoproteins, and iron. Astonishingly, an ounce of semen has the same value as sixty ounces of blood, in terms of the vital elements it provides. Dr Frederick McCann agrees that semen has a great potential for enhancing life and health, as some ancient traditions also believed.[3]

However, it is not clear why semen has such a high concentration of valuable body chemicals if its main function is to transport sperm. An ounce of semen has the same amount of the most important chemicals as sixty ounces of blood. The brain and the semen have similar levels of lecithin, cholesterol, and phosphorus. The semen also has more fructose, citric acid, spermine, and prostaglandins than other tissues. Moreover, the semen has more zinc, ascorbic acid, inositol, glyceryl, phosphorylcholine, and free amino acids than most tissues. For example, it has 33 times more neutral amino acids, 28 times more acidic amino acids, and 57 times more basic amino acids than blood. This suggests that women may benefit from absorbing body chemicals from male semen, besides prostaglandins, and improve their health and well-being. On the other hand, a man may conserve and use these valuable body chemicals for himself, by practising a moderate sexual lifestyle and boosting his brain and body vitality.

Modern psychology often considers sexual restraint as unhealthy for the mind and body, but it ignores the fact that many great thinkers and artists of the past and present were celibates. This is not to say that celibacy is the only way to live but to challenge the modern view that it is unnatural or harmful. The semen is a valuable fluid that contains substances that nourish the brain and nervous system. If women can benefit from absorbing semen from men during sex, then men can also benefit from keeping their semen in their bodies. On the other hand, losing semen can weaken the body and brain, and deprive them of substances like lecithin, which can help treat nervous disorders caused by sexual excess. It has been shown that women can get some of these substances from men during sex, but it may also be true that men can use these substances for their own mental and physical development if they do not waste them in sex. Interestingly, the semen and the brain have a similar chemical makeup, more than any other tissues in the body.[4] Many physiological evidences show the value of continence, such as:

- The semen and the central nervous system have a similar chemical composition, both being rich in lecithin, cholesterol and phosphorus compounds, which means that losing semen can take away substances that are needed for the nutrition of the nervous tissues.

- Losing semen voluntarily (through masturbation, coitus, coitus interruptus, and contraceptive methods) or involuntarily (through nocturnal emissions, diurnal emissions, spermatorrhea, etc.) can harm and weaken the body and brain.

- The sexual orgasm can temporarily drain the nervous system, and if done too often can lead to chronic nerve weakness (sexual neurasthenia).

- Continence can benefit the brain (because the lecithin from the semen is a good brain food). This is why some of the greatest intellectual geniuses in history were celibates, such as Pythagoras, Plato, Aristotle, Leonardo da Vinci, Spinoza, Newton, Kant, Beethoven, Herbert Spencer, etc.

- Recent physiological evidence, showing that semen contains substances of great physiological value (such as Poehl's Spermine, which is a nerve-stimulant, lecithin, cholesterol, vitamin E, male sex hormones, etc.) supports the idea that continence is beneficial to health, as do the experiments of Prof. Brown-Sequard on the vitalizing effects of testicular extracts and those of Prof. Steinach on the rejuvenation that follows the forced conservation of semen through tying the efferent testicular duct.

- Many experts in physiology, urology, genito-urinary diseases, neurology, psychiatry, sexology, gynaecology and endocrinology agree on the physiological value of continence. Some of these authorities are Moll, Kraepelin, Marshall, Lydston, Talmey and others.[5]

Dr. Jacobson asked two hundred professors of physiology, hygiene, venereal diseases, nervous diseases, neurology and psychiatry about their opinions on continence. Almost all of them said that continence is good for health. Here are some of their answers. Many experts in medicine, psychology, and sexology have stated that sexual continence, or abstaining from sex, is not harmful, but rather beneficial, for young men and their health. They have also pointed out the advantages of continence in preventing venereal diseases. Some of the quotes from these experts are:

- Kraepelin: "Continence is not injurious, and its advantages in avoiding venereal infection are apparent."

- Gaertner: "Continence is not injurious to young men."

- Gramer: "Sexual continence before marriage is not injurious."

- Finkler: "Sexual continence is not injurious to young men, but, on the contrary, is beneficial to body and mind."

- Lassar: "Sexual continence is not injurious to young men."

- Seifert: "My experience teaches me that continence is not injurious."

- Gruber: "There is no reason why continence should be injurious."

- Jurgensen: "Sexual continence is not injurious."

- Strumpell: "Continence is indirectly useful in preventing venereal infection, and is not injurious."

- Hoffman: "Sexual continence is useful."

- Tuczek: "Continence is beneficial."

- Von Leyden: "I have never seen injurious consequences from continence."

- Hein: "In most men sexual continence is not injurious."

- Von Grutzner: "Sexual continence is rarely injurious."

- Meschede: "I have never seen a case of insanity caused by sexual continence."

- Weber: "Continence is not injurious to young men, but, on the contrary, is useful."

- Hoche: "Sexual continence is not injurious to young men and does not lead to masturbation."

- Neisser: "Most of our young men could remain continent much longer than in the case nowadays."

- Aschffenberg: "Even those who are predisposed to nervousness do not suffer any harm from sexual continence if the impression is awakened in them that abstinence can never be injurious."

- Moll: "At present, most medical men agree that sexual abstinence, in a general way, is not harmful."

- Hutchinson: "The belief that the exercise of the sex function is necessary to the health of the male at any age is a pure delusion while before full maturity it is highly injurious."[6]

Some of the eminent authorities on sex who support the view that sexual continence is harmless and beneficial to health are Forel, Moll, Montegazza, Fournier, Dubois, Furbringer, Loewenfeld, Krafft-Ebing, Lydston, Ruggles, Oesterling, Chassaignac, Beale, Ribbing, Acton, Hegar, Marshall, Robinowitch, Spitzka, Talmey, Sajous, Bruce, Brown-Sequard, and others.

Professor Von Gruber of Munich, a renowned European expert on sex, wrote in his article "The Hygienic Significance of Marriage" that it is absurd to compare semen to urine, which needs to be expelled regularly, but rather to a vital fluid that is reabsorbed during sexual continence, and that this reabsorption has a positive effect on the physiological system, as shown by the large number of intellectual geniuses who were celibates.

Let's know more about medical, psychological, and sexological authorities who have said that sexual continence, or not having sex, is good, not bad, for young men and their health. They have also mentioned the benefits of continence in avoiding venereal diseases. Here are some of their quotes:[7]

- Talmey: "Without sexual stimulation, the semen and sperm are produced less and resorbed fully by the seminal vesicles, making continence easy and natural. Keeping this vital fluid, he says, is needed for the best strength of body and mind, while losing it is bad. A man can live his whole life in complete continence, without harm, but only with benefit, as shown by such men as Leonardo da Vinci, Kant, Beethoven, Spencer, etc."

- Dubois: "Sexual excess, not continence, causes neurasthenia, unlike what the Freudian school wrongly says."

- Fournier: "The idea of 'the dangers of continence for the young man' is ridiculous, and in his years of medical practice, he has never seen one such case."

- Montegazza: "Chastity has benefits for the body and the brain."

- Kellogg: "Many of the famous Greek athletes of the past (as Astylos, Dopompos and others mentioned by Plato) were continent during their training, which made them very strong."

- Furbringer: "Sexual continence is not injurious to health as is commonly believed, according to the medical profession." He also writes: "Neurasthenia in an unmarried person is usually due to masturbation or some other kind of lust."

- Krafft-Ebing: "The 'diseases of abstinence' are a myth."

- Loewenfeld: "A sexually normal person can live in permanent continence without any ill-effects."

- Lydston: "Continence itself is probably never harmful. The retention of the seminal secretion in the testes often leads to great bodily and mental vigor." He also says: "One can be perfectly healthy and physically strong while leading a life of absolute continence."

- Ruggles: "Sexual abstinence is good for health and increases vitality through resorption of the semen."

- Perier: "The idea of the imaginary dangers of sexual continence is false, and it is a 'physical, moral and mental protection for young men'."

- Rohleder: "The advice of doctors who suggest sexual intercourse to young men is dishonest."

- Chassaignac: "The healthier the person, the easier to be completely abstinent; only the sick and neurotic person finds it hard to do so."

- Oesterling: "One should say again and again that abstinence and the most absolute purity are in harmony with the laws of physiology and morality, and that sexual indulgence is not more justified by physiology and psychology than by morality and religion."

- Beale: "No man has ever been harmed by sexual abstinence when he has practised it."

- Ribbing: "I have seen many young men who have lived in total continence without any trouble or harm."

- Clarke: "Continence improves health and energy, while incontinence does the opposite."

- Surbled: "The harms of incontinence are clear and undeniable; those caused by continence are imaginary."

- Acton: "The common idea that abstinence makes the genital organs shrink and causes impotence is a serious mistake. Chastity does not hurt the body or the soul."

- Hegar: "The 'sexual necessity' myth is a delusion, while Ribbing, another distinguished gynaecologist, emphasizes the need for sexual discipline and continence."

- Marshall: "In his 'Introduction to Sex Physiology', he shows the need for such control over the reproductive function and the transformation of sex energy into higher mental forms of expression, as was the case with many intellectual geniuses of the past, who were celibates."

- Robinowitch: "Sexual continence is not only harmless but beneficial."[8]

American Medicine, in its editorial of July 1, 1905, says, "It should not be hard to persuade any mature man that continence can be a normal state of civilized man." In 1906, the American Medical Association agreed that "continence is not harmful to health". The International Brussels Congress also stated that a chaste life for a man is not bad for health, but, on the contrary, can be advised from a purely hygienic point of view. The congress said, "Most of the great medical thinkers agree that it is not bad for the health of a man to keep his body clean". The medical faculty of Christiania University declared: "The claim that a chaste life will be bad for health is not based on our unanimous experience. We have no evidence of any harm from a pure and moral life".[9] There is strong evidence of the benefits of continence and that the supposed "sexual necessity" is an illusion from the study of the weakening effects of sexual orgasm, which are immediate and noticeable.

CHAPTER VI

Nourishing Properties of Semen as Per Ayurveda

One drop of semen in manufactured out of forty drops of blood according to modern medical science. According to Ayurveda, it is elaborated out of eighty drops of blood.[10] Ayurveda, an ancient system of medicine from India, semen is the final product of a complex process of tissue transformation that starts from food. This process was first described by Ācharya Sushruta, a pioneer of surgery and anatomy, around 600 BC.

He explained that food, after digestion, becomes chyle, a milky fluid that carries nutrients. Chyle, in five days, becomes blood, the liquid tissue that circulates in the body. Blood, in another five days, becomes flesh, the solid tissue that forms the muscles and organs. Flesh, in five more days, becomes fat, the oily tissue that lubricates the joints and skin. Fat, in another five days, becomes bone, the hard tissue that supports the skeleton. Bone, in five more days, becomes bone marrow, the soft tissue that fills the bone cavities. And finally, bone marrow, in the last five days, becomes semen, the reproductive tissue that carries the sperm. The same process occurs in women, where the final product is the ovum, the female reproductive cell. The whole process takes about 30 days to complete.[11]

Modern science, on the other hand, has a different view of semen formation and composition. According to scientists, semen is a mixture of sperm and seminal fluid, which are produced by the testes and accessory glands in the male reproductive system. The sperm are the male reproductive cells that carry the genetic material. The seminal fluid is a liquid that provides nourishment, protection, and motility to the sperm.

The entire process of spermatogenesis typically lasts for an average duration of 74 days.[12] consequently, the process of sperm cell maturation within the testes' incubating chamber typically spans approximately two months.

Following the maturation process, sperm cells are expelled into the epididymis. The process of sperm maturation in the epididymis requires an additional 14 days. This implies that it takes approximately three months for the entire cycle to be completed. Seminal fluid exhibits distinct characteristics. This chemical is easily accessible as it is supplied every two days. Despite its faster production, it still requires resources for replenishment. During these processes, your body is expending energy by converting glycogen and fructose. This is in addition to the energy needed to produce the hormonal messages that are necessary to initiate the processes in the first place.

Consequently, the process of replenishing sperm takes more time compared to replenishing seminal fluid. This may explain why some individuals mistakenly believe that sperm cannot be depleted. Indeed, it is feasible to experience ejaculation with a substantial volume of seminal fluid, despite having a diminished number or subpar quality of sperm. It is indeed possible to exhaust your sperm supply.[13]

Semen production is an automatic biological process in our bodies, but we often do not appreciate its value. Semen contains immense energy and potential in every drop. One drop of semen can create many great personalities, such as heroes, scientists, warriors, and writers. And many more great personalities will continue to be born from one drop of semen. This is an undeniable truth.

CHAPTER VII

Why Brahmacharya is Not a Danger, But a Blessing

Many people today believe that continence, or sexual abstinence, is harmful to health and happiness and that it is a relic of old-fashioned religious dogma and scientific ignorance. Some self-proclaimed experts on sexuality have used this belief to sell their books and products, and have created a fear of continence among the public, who think that it can cause nervous and mental disorders and pose a serious health risk. Some doctors and psychoanalysts have also adopted this view, and have advised young men to have sex with prostitutes and expose themselves to venereal diseases, rather than face the supposed hazards of abstinence. However, this view is not based on sound evidence, but on false assumptions and prejudices.

A careful examination of the facts will show that continence is not only harmless, but beneficial for the physical and mental well-being of the individual and that when problems arise in someone who is not having normal sexual relations, the cause is not continence, but some other form of sexual expression, such as masturbation, excessive nocturnal emissions, etc. It is well known that semen contains many substances that are vital for the nourishment and functioning of the nervous system and the brain, such as lecithin, cholesterol, phosphorus, and others. Therefore, it is logical to conclude that continence, or the conservation of semen, means the conservation of these substances and the enhancement of vitality, while incontinence, or the loss of semen, means the loss of these substances and the reduction of vitality. Moreover, chronic loss of semen can lead to the symptoms of old age, which some scientists have tried to reverse by increasing the amount of sex hormones in the blood.

Mark Jacua's *Conservation Therapy* explains sex hormones are produced by the sex glands, both internally and externally, and are present in the semen. They are responsible for the physical and mental characteristics of the individual. Men have much higher levels of testosterone, the main male sex hormone, than women. Testosterone affects not only the body, but also the brain, and has a stimulating effect on the mind. It has been shown that testosterone is related to intelligence, aggression, motivation, energy, and mood in both men and women.

Testosterone levels decrease in men who are castrated, either by accident or disease, and they experience a decline in energy, mood, and motivation. These effects can be reversed by administering testosterone. Men who have inactive testes also have low energy levels, which depend on the amount of testosterone they receive. Their energy levels increase after receiving testosterone and decrease until the next dose. Lack of testosterone in men who have reached puberty results in a condition called "eunuchoidism", which is marked by apathy, withdrawal, depression, lack of initiative, and hypoactivity.[14] Testosterone is a sex hormone that affects the brain and may explain why men have historically achieved more than women in mental fields. Even today, with more opportunities for women, men still get 98% of all patents. Progesterone, the main female sex hormone, is linked to mood, but not to intelligence. Testosterone has been shown to improve spatial ability in men, but only if it is present in enough amounts during a key developmental stage 2.[15]

Testosterone levels are low in men with severe mental disorders, such as schizophrenia, psychosis, and anorexia nervosa. These men (and women) also have more sexual activity. Kraemer (1967) found that less sexual activity in men increases testosterone levels, which may boost IQ, mood, and motivation. In some schizophrenics, more sexual activity precedes episodes. This suggests that more sexual activity may worsen severe mental problems.[16]

Testosterone levels also control prostaglandin levels in the body. Prostaglandins are substances that are made and used in many parts of the body. They have the strongest effects of any natural substances on living tissue. They are involved in many body functions, such as blood pressure, pain, inflammation, and nerve signals. They may also affect serotonin levels in the brain since serotonin and prostaglandins have similar effects.[17]

Most animals do not make prostaglandins, even though their biochemistry is similar to humans. Only rabbits, sheep, and some monkeys make prostaglandins, and humans make much more than them. The male seminal vesicles make the most prostaglandins in the body, and male semen has a lot of prostaglandins.

Men lose more prostaglandins in one ejaculation than women make in their whole body in a day. It is not clear why male semen has prostaglandins since they do not help sperm or fertilization. Women absorb male prostaglandins after sex in the vagina and uterus, and they have special cells in the uterus to receive them. There is an old saying that women get stronger than men during sex, and this may be true on a chemical level. Prostaglandins are one of the most refined products of the body, and women get these "super-chemicals" from men.[18]

CHAPTER VIII

The Harmful Effects of Sexual Orgasm

Sexual orgasm is often seen as a source of pleasure and satisfaction, but it can also have negative consequences for health and well-being. There is convincing evidence that sexual continence, or abstaining from sex, is beneficial and that the supposed "sexual necessity" is a myth. This evidence comes from the study of the debilitating effects of sexual orgasm, which are immediate and severe. These effects are not only due to the nervous system, but also to the loss of semen, which contains calcium, lecithin, and other substances that are essential for the normal functioning of the nerves.

Havelock Ellis, in his "Studies in the Psychology of Sex", cites the observations of Dr. F.B. Robinson on this topic, as reported in the New York State Medical Journal. He notes that some animals, such as stallions, bulls, and boars, experience fainting, exhaustion, or even death after their first sexual intercourse, which Robinson attributes to brain anemia caused by the loss of semen. He also mentions a case of a mare dying right after mating. Dogs, however, do not faint, because their sexual intercourse is longer and less shocking; also, they do not have seminal vesicles, which store semen.[19]

Havelock Ellis writes: "When we have realized how profound the organic convulsion is involved in the process of detumescence, and how great the motor excitement involved, we can understand how it is that very serious effects may follow coitus. Even in animals, this is sometimes the case. Young bulls and stallions have fallen into a faint after the first congress; boars may be seriously affected similarly; mares have been known even to fall dead. In the human species, and especially men, probably, as Bryan Robinson remarks, because women are protected by the greater slowness with which detumescence occurs in them - not only death itself but innumerable disorders and accidents have been known to follow immediately after coitus, these results being mainly due to the vascular and muscular excitement involved in the process of detumescence. Fainting, vomiting, urination, and defecation have been noted as occurring in young men after the first coitus.

Epilepsy has been not frequently recorded. Lesions of various organs, even rupture of the spleen, have sometimes taken place. In men of mature age, the arteries have at times been unable to resist the high blood pressure and cerebral haemorrhage with paralysis has occurred. In elderly men, the excitement of intercourse with a strange woman has sometimes caused death, and various cases are known of eminent persons who have thus died in the arms of young wives or prostitutes."[20]

He also refers to several cases of men dying after sexual intercourse with women who were not their wives, such as the famous Russian general Skobeloff, a judge, a man of seventy, a man of forty-eight, a young man, and a man of sixty. These deaths usually happen in older men, and usually after sex with unfamiliar women, which is more intense and violent than with their wives. He also mentions the case of Atilla, the king of the Huns, who died while having sex with his young wife.

Acton, a respected medical expert, notes that some people have a seizure-like spasm at the end of the orgasm. This makes them very tired. This is very obvious in male-female and this also happens in other animals. The link between reproduction and death is well-known in flying insects, such as the common mayfly. They become winged, dance and mate, lay eggs and die, all in a few hours. "In higher animals", these authors say, "the risk of dying from reproduction has become much smaller, but death may still happen, even in human life, as the direct result of love. The tiring effect of even a little sexual activity is well known, as well as the higher chance of getting sick when the person's energy is low. Reproduction is the start of death."[21]

In his book, "Science Discovered the Physiological Benefits of Continence," RW Bernard highlights the essential functions of the sexual apparatus. There are two main functions: Internal Secretion, which is primary, and Reproduction, which is secondary. Any misuse of these endocrine organs can lead to nervous disorders, premature ageing, and even death.

Bernard quotes Melville Keith, M.D., in "The Marriage Law," stating that with every emission of semen, valuable nutrients and blood corpuscles are lost. This loss impacts the body's ability to form essential substances like joint oil, new muscles, and brain material. Keith emphasizes that expelling semen leads to a waste of life's vital components, causing negative consequences such as paralysis, palsy, apoplexy, rheumatism, and other health issues.[22]

The similarity between a sexual orgasm and an epileptic attack is noted by various authors. The sudden withdrawal of calcium during a seminal discharge biochemically triggers tetany-like symptoms, resembling an epileptic attack. According to Acton, the mental dullness and physical exhaustion following a sexual orgasm mirror the effects of an epileptic attack. Acton emphasizes that only mature individuals can handle occasional acts of copulation without causing harm, especially in young individuals where conserving vital powers for growth and development is crucial.[23]

Dr. Deslandes noticed that after engaging in sexual activity, some individuals, like Napoleon, experience epileptic attacks. He explains that certain people prone to epilepsy may have seizures when involved in sexual intercourse. This connection is highlighted through the example of Napoleon, who suffered seizures whenever he attempted copulation.[24]

In his work "Sanity and Insanity," English psychiatrist Mercier discusses the aftermath of sexual activity. He mentions that the exhaustion and fatigue following coitus indicate a significant strain on the body's energy, primarily affecting the nervous system and the brain. While a normally constituted organism can handle the stress of the sexual orgasm unless repeated excessively, those with naturally lower energy levels may experience disturbed cerebral functioning, especially if such indulgence begins at an early age.

Mercier notes that a portion of insanity cases is attributed to sexual excess, leading to a deterioration of the nervous system's higher powers.[25] According to Mercier, the sexual orgasm inherently has a disintegrative influence on the organism, causing energy loss and resulting in apathy, lethargy, and dementia, particularly when frequently repeated. This reduced energy in the nervous system leads to a lack of manifestations or feeble expressions of energy.

Mercier describes this condition as dementia, characterized by the inability to perform mental operations, dullness, slowness of feeling, and the loss of higher emotions. Even in cases of less excessive indulgence, there is degradation, and deterioration resembles dementia, indicating a deficiency in stored energy.[26]

Mercier also mentions a significant number of individuals who experience premature mental power decay, energy exhaustion, and senility due to excessive sexual indulgence in early life. Young individuals, initially energetic, engage in sexual excesses that may seem harmless at the time. However, as time passes, the consequences become evident, likened to a spendthrift living on his capital, exhausting sexual energy prematurely and facing the repercussions before middle age.[27]

Herbert Spender, a wise philosopher who lived a celibate life, explains the consequences of too much sexual activity. He notes that it can lead to chronic health issues, reduced physical activity, a decline in mental power, and sometimes even insanity. Specialists, who can evaluate well, agree that the overall harm from such excesses surpasses that from all other types of excess combined.[28]

Havelock Ellis, discussing a case in the "Journal of Mental Science" from January 1879, mentions a man whose three wives became insane after marriage due to sexual excess. He describes cases where physical exhaustion, suspicions, and delusions are common outcomes of sexual excess. Hutchinson, as noted in the Archives of Surgery in January 1893, records three cases of temporary blindness in men resulting from sexual excess after marriage. Historical medical sources also attribute various adverse effects to coitus, such as insanity, syncope, epilepsy, loss of memory, blindness, baldness, unilateral perspiration, and even death.[29]

Professor Lydston points out that the consequences of sexual excess are similar to those of masturbation. Both stem from the disturbance of blood chemistry and general metabolism caused by the removal of substances like calcium, phosphorus, lecithin, cholesterol, albumen, and iron, which are components of semen. While attention has been more focused on the negative effects of masturbation, Lydston believes that sexual excess is a significant cause of neurasthenia, a widespread modern disease. He emphasizes that moderation in sexual intercourse not only promotes prolonged virility but also contributes to longevity. Many cases of neurasthenia, in both males and females, are attributed to sexual excess.[30]

Dr Talmey explains that frequently engaging in sexual activity directly leads to anemia, malnutrition, weakened muscles and nerves, and mental exhaustion. People who indulge in sexual excess can be identified by their pale, long, and flabby faces with tense features. They often feel melancholic and are generally not suitable for strenuous or prolonged physical or mental work. Their ability to resist illnesses is low, and many women's health declines after a certain period of married life due to the same reason.[31]

Professor Von Gruber, while uncertain about the claim that sexual abstinence may harm the nervous system, is certain that sexual excess does. He believes that frequent semen discharges result in a "reduction of the peculiar internal secretion of the testes," normally absorbed into the bloodstream. The immediate effects of sexual excess include depression, fatigue, and exhaustion. Additional symptoms comprise lumbar pressure, nervous irritability, head pressure, dullness, insomnia, ringing in the ears, spots before the eyes, light aversion, weak trembling, actual shaking, heart palpitations, a tendency to sweat, and muscle weakness.

Memory weakens, neurasthenia sets in, melancholic depression occurs, and there is a reluctance to engage in physical or mental efforts. Digestive activity becomes less efficient, and food utilization decreases. The blood becomes deficient, leading to lowered resistance to infectious bacteria, particularly the tubercle bacillus.

Sexual excess is known to predispose to consumption due to its tendency to drain the body of calcium. Genital weakness, premature ejaculation, frequent nocturnal emissions, and increasing impotence are common. The more frequent nocturnal emissions exacerbate nervous irritability and exhaustion, especially in the young and the elderly. In the young, sexual excess hinders physical and mental development by negatively affecting metabolism and growth processes. In the elderly, it hastens death, often causing heart failure.[32]

CHAPTER IX

The Myth of Masturbation as Need For Humanity

This chapter aims to help you see masturbation in a new light, free from the misconceptions that might have clouded your understanding. Dr. El Lernanto discusses how nerve exhaustion shows up in males through spermatorrhea, an involuntary release of semen. This can occur due to sexual and other passionate activities, both inside and outside of marital relations, affecting both adults and youths.[33]

The connection between the genitals and the head is crucial. Two common issues, masturbation and onanism (congressus interruptus of Onan), often lead to general breakdowns more than excesses in regular sexual activities. Among these, masturbation is riskier as it usually starts in immature children and, when done excessively, causes fatigue and exhaustion in the central nervous system.

Dr Bernard Talmey suggests that neurasthenia results from lecithin starvation in nerve cells due to sexual lecithin withdrawals. This is highlighted in his paper, "Sexual Problems of Today, with a Case of Hysterical Insanity Caused by Excessive Masturbation."[34]

In 1772, Wichman observed a link between spermatorrhea, consumption, and hypochondria. He believed that masturbation and excessive sexual activity were predisposing factors, with constipation playing an exciting role. Thin, pale, and enervated men, especially those lazy in actions, could be suspected of these causes.[35]

Celsus and Satorius also linked seminal losses to consumption and other health issues, emphasizing the impact on the body. Miescher breaks down the tail of the spermatozoon like this:[36]

- Protein: 41.90%

- Phosphorized fats (lecithin): 31.83%

- Cholesterin: 26.27%

Considering the entire spermatozoon, here's the composition:[37]

- Protein: 83.76%

- Lecithin: 7.47%

- Other fats: 4.53%

- Cholesterin: 2.53%

Chakraberty adds to this by describing the tail as made up of proteins, lecithin, cholesterin, and lipoids. He points out that its composition is similar to non-medullated nerves or the axis-cylinder.[38]

When sex glands withdraw too many lipoids from the blood, it affects the adrenal cortex, much like how Miescher observed the withdrawal of protein impacting the muscles. This over activity in the gonads, taking away lipoids from the adrenal cortex, leads to its atrophy.[39]

In cases of dementia praecox, commonly found in habitual masturbators, Mott observed not only the atrophy of the adrenal cortex but also progressive shrinkage of the testicles. Additionally, withdrawing nucleoproteins and other substances excessively from the blood to create spermatozoa can result in the reduction of the thymus gland's size and its subsequent atrophy. This might explain why such changes often occur after puberty.[40]

Considering the richness of lecithin in the pineal gland, one might wonder if the atrophy of the pineal gland, accompanying that of the thymus, is due to a similar cause. Prof. Sajous points out the remarkable richness of nucleins in thymic tissue and lymphocytes, similar to the heads of the spermatozoan.[41]

CHAPTER X

The Surprising Connection between Brain and Semen

Similarities between Brain Cells and Spermatozoa

The proteins found in brain cells and the heads of spermatozoa share striking similarities. Both contain abundant nucleic acid and the heads of spermatozoa, like the Nissl substance in brain cells, are rich in nucleoproteins. The general formation of both spermatozoa and cortical brain cells is remarkably alike. Notably, spermatozoa, in each ejaculation releasing a whopping 226 million, lose a considerable amount of phosphorus, second only to brain cells in the body.[42]

Varieties of Brain Lipoids and Their Impact

Brain lipoids come in two types. Some, like lecithin, exist in other organs, while others, such as cephalin, phrenosin, and keratin, are exclusive to the brain. The white matter of the brain contains double the cholesterin compared to the grey matter. In contrast, the grey matter boasts double the lecithin and triple the cephalin. This explains why, as observed by Lassaigne, the amount of fat and lecithin in the brain decreases significantly in insane subjects.[43]

Biochemical Relationship (Semen & Nervous System)

Lecithin and cholesterin are key components in the active protoplasm of nerve and brain cells, as well as in semen, which shares similarities with the brain as a fatty substance. This highlights a significant biochemical connection, through the blood, between semen and the central nervous system. According to Sajous, lecithin is prominent in various body parts, including the brain, nerves, yolk of egg, semen, pus, white blood corpuscles, and the electrical organs of the ray.[44]

Spermatozoa and Cerebral Cortex Cells

The existence of an intimate relationship between spermatozoa and cells in the cerebral cortex is evident. If spermatozoa aren't discharged, they may be reabsorbed into the bloodstream and transported to the brain. In their chemical composition and elongated form, they resemble brain cells, both lacking the ability to reproduce, unlike most other cells. This connection could potentially extend to the mobile neuroglia in the brain and spinal marrow.[45]

Phosphorus Metabolism and Thinking

Dr. Evans suggests an intriguing idea that thinking is a phase of phosphorus metabolism in the brain. During mental exertion, phosphates increase in excreta, indicating the oxidation of phosphorus compounds in the brain. Phosphorus, oxygen, and sufficient thyroid hormone are crucial for normal brain electricity generation. Deficiency in any of these elements leads to deficient brain action.[46]

Semen Loss and Neurasthenia

Neurasthenia, a condition of phosphorus or lecithin deficiency, may result from excessive semen loss. Lecithin, abundant in semen, plays a crucial role in maintaining nerve vitality. The action of alcohol and sexual excess, both removing lecithin from the brain, can lead to neuropsychopathic conditions and even insanity.[47]

Semen Preservation for Brain Health

Prof. Eugen Steinach's experiments show that internal secretions from sex glands, once resorbed into circulation, primarily reach the brain and spinal cord, where they are stored. Steinach's findings suggest that these secretions influence the central nervous system, potentially inducing local changes in blood supply and affecting various body parts.[48]

CHAPTER XI

A Cross-Cultural Study of Depression and Sexuality

A Hidden Connection Many of us do not realize how much our physical and mental health are intertwined. In this section, we will examine how losing semen can affect the brain, and how different sexual attitudes in developed countries relate to depression rates.

We will reveal the connection between sexual practices and mental wellness, especially in cultures that support both sexual openness and celibacy. We aim to shed light on a topic that is often taboo in society.

We will investigate the scientific evidence and compare the common beliefs with the actual effects of semen retention on the brain. We hope to foster awareness, empathy, and mental strength in the face of changing social norms.

Think about the subtle link between our physical and mental aspects, and look for clues in depression data where sexual expression and abstinence affect mental health on a large scale.

Delving into Global Statistics and Root Causes[49]

Nowadays, Problems of depression, sadness, loss of interest, guilt, sleeping disorders, poor concentration, tiredness, anxiety & fear have become common in youth. Depression, also known as major depressive disorder, is a mental health disorder that negatively affects how a person feels, thinks, and acts. What is interesting to note is that India being a land of spirituality, is standing nowhere, whether the case of the high frequency of depression or low frequency of depression, which has been appended in the statists below. Let's first have a look at the symptoms of depression.

Symptoms of depression

Varied in intensity, depression exhibits a range of symptoms. And include the following:

- A persistent feeling of sadness

- Loss of interest in activities once enjoyed

- Changes in appetite – weight loss or gain

- Trouble sleeping or sleeping too much

- Loss of energy or increased fatigue

- Increase in purposeless tasks or physical activities such as pacing

- Slowed movements and speech

- Feeling guilty or worthless

- Difficulty thinking or concentrating

- Decreased confidence and self-esteem

- Negative, bleak, or pessimistic attitude

- Self-harmful or suicidal thoughts or actions

About 1 in 15 adults experience depression each year, and 1 in 6 people will go through depression at some point. An Our World in Data study estimates about 3.4% (2-6% when including the margin of error) of the global population has depression. This is about 264 million people worldwide. According to WHO estimates, the ten countries with the highest prevalence of depression are:

Top 10 Countries with the Highest Rates of Depression

1. Ukraine - 6.3%

2. United States - 5.9% (tie)

3. Estonia - 5.9% (tie)

4. Australia - 5.9% (tie)

5. Brazil - 5.8%

6. Greece - 5.7% (tie)

7. Portugal - 5.7% (tie)

8. Belarus - 5.6% (tie)

9. Finland - 5.6% (tie)

10. Lithuania - 5.6% (tie)

Top 10 Countries with the Lowest Rates of Depression

1. Solomon Islands - 2.9%

2. Papua New Guinea - 3.0% (tie)

3. Timor-Leste - 3.0% (tie)

4. Vanuatu - 3.1% (tie)

5. Kiribati - 3.1% (tie)

6. Tonga - 3.2% (tie)

7. Samoa - 3.2% (tie)

8. Laos - 3.2% (tie)

9. Nepal - 3.2% (tie)

10. Philippines - 3.3%

While the numbers listed above (and below) are valuable and vital, it is important to remember that the actual rates are likely much higher, especially in less developed countries. Depression is much more likely to be diagnosed in highly developed countries, with more robust healthcare infrastructures better equipped to identify and treat mental illnesses.

Therefore, less developed countries do not necessarily have less depression—rather, their treatment of mental illnesses often takes a back seat to broader concerns such as hunger, disease, and sanitation. The World Health Organization estimates that 76–85% of people with mental disorders in low-and middle-income countries don't have the needed treatment. Moreover, even in developed nations, many cases of mental illness go undiagnosed and unreported because the patients are either ashamed or unaware that it's a medically treatable condition.

How common is depression?

More than 264 million people suffer from depression worldwide. (World Health Organization, 2020)

- Depression reigns as the top global cause of disability. (World Health Organization, 2020)

- Neuropsychiatric disorders top the list of disabilities in the U.S., with major depressive disorder being the most common. (National Institute of Mental Health, 2013)

Depression Statistics in America

- As per the National Institute of Mental Health (2017), around 17.[3] million adults (7.1% of the adult population) have encountered a major depressive episode.

- As the National Institute of Mental Health (2017) indicated, 63.8% of adults and 70.77% of adolescents with major depressive episodes experienced severe impairment.

- Centres for Disease Control (2017) has reported women are almost twice as likely as men to suffer from depression.

- In 2017, the National Institute of Mental Health found that adults (11.3%) and adolescents (16.9%) identifying with multiple races had the highest rates of major depressive episodes.

Depression statistics by age

- According to the Substance Abuse and Mental Health Services Association (2018), teens aged 12 to 17 had the greatest price of significant depressive episodes (14.4%) complied with young people matured 18 to 25 (13.8%).

- As per the 2018 Substance Abuse and Mental Health Services Association report, older adults aged 50 andabove exhibited the lowest occurrence of major depressive episodes, with a rate of 4.5%.

- As of 2018, 11.[5] million adult adults experienced a major depressive episode with severe impairment. (Substance Abuse and Mental Health Services Association, 2018).

- From 2013 to 2018, the rate of severe depression among college students increased from 9.4% to 21,1%. (Journal of Adolescent Health 2019).

- From 2007 to 2018, the rate of depression ranging from moderate to severe increased from 23,2% to 41,1%. (Journal of Adolescent Health 2019).

Mental Health Statistics at Global Level As Per Forbes

- 21% of U.S. adults experienced a mental health condition in 2020.

- 5.6% of U.S. adults experienced a serious mental health condition in 2020, which is often defined as a psychotic disorder, bipolar disorder or a severe anxiety or eating disorder that significantly impairs functioning.

- In 2020, 32.1% of U.S. adults experienced both a mental health condition and substance abuse.

- In 2019, 15.3% of U.S. veterans experienced a mental health condition, such as post-traumatic stress disorder (PTSD), depression or substance abuse

- As of 2020, suicide is the second leading cause of death for U.S. children ages 10 to 14, preceded only by unintentional injury.

- The impact depression and anxiety has on the global economy can be measured in $1 trillion in lost productivity each year.

- Young adults ages 18 to 25 in the U.S have the highest rate of experiencing any mental health concerns (30.6%) compared to adults aged 26 to 49 years, and the highest rate of serious mental illness (9.7%).

(Nationally: In 2020, 21% of U.S. adults (52.9 million) experienced a mental health condition)

  - Young adults ages 18 to 25 in the U.S have the highest rate of experiencing mental health conditions (30.6%), followed by those ages 26 to 49 (25.3%) and adults ages 50 and over (14.5%).

  - The majority of youth (70%) in juvenile detention centers have been diagnosed with a mental health disorder.

  - Severe mental health conditions cost the U.S. Economy $193.[2] billion in lost revenue.

The Rise of Depression among Young People

Many young people, aged 12 to 25, struggle with various forms of depression. Some of the main causes are premarital sex, free sex, the legality of pornography, excessive sex promotion, and a lack of moral and cultural education. These factors are becoming more common in the lifestyle of many countries, except India.

A recent report by the Heritage Center for Data Analysis examined the link between teenage sexual activity and emotional health. Using data from the National Longitudinal Survey of Adolescent Health, the authors compared the levels of happiness, depression, and suicide attempts among sexually active and non-sexually active adolescents, controlling for demographic and family factors. The report found that sexually active adolescents were significantly less happy, more depressed, and more likely to attempt suicide than their non-sexually active peers. The report also suggested that abstinence education programs could help promote the delay of sexual activity and the development of healthy relationships among teenagers as Sexually Active Teenagers Are More Likely to Be Depressed and To Attempt Suicide.[50]

The Role of Hindu Culture and Brahmacharya

India (Bharat) has not experienced the same high levels of mental distress as other countries. However, it is important to note that cultural and Brahmacharya Education disappeared from the education system in 1835 due to the English Education Act. We should thank the Spiritual Masters, Yogis, and Gurus in India who stress the importance of Hindu Culture and Brahmacharya for mental strength. The culture of a country affects the mental health of its people and the availability of mental health care services. Moreover, some depression symptoms are more common in certain cultures due to cultural factors.

Mental disorders are spreading fast across the world. It is vital to tackle this problem by promoting the core science of Vedic Education along with modern scientific knowledge and practical research.

CHAPTER XII

Unveiling The Harmful Effects of Too Much Self-Pleasure

In my six-year of social awareness journey, talking to millions of followers, I've seen various practical issues that happen when people engage in too much self-pleasure out of Masturbation. This section talks about the real problems faced by those who've gone down this road, shining a light on how it affects their physical and mental health.

Practical Consequences:

- Confidence takes a nosedive, and the person is left confused about why it's happening.

- Important parts of semen are wasted, making it more like water.

- Once energetic bodies and minds become worn out, like a battery running out, due to lust and semen loss.

- People start questioning what to do, even when they have guidance, leading to repeated indecision.

- Eyesight weakens, facial glow fades, positive qualities diminish, and overall personality takes a hit.

- Weakness in semen glands causes premature ejaculation triggered by just seeing, thinking, or touching the opposite sex.

- Erectile dysfunction causes problems in marriage, infertility, and eventually,

- Semen is released before and after urination, urine becomes frothy, and there's a strange taste on the tongue.

- Semen release due to loud noises and lifting light weights.

- Sleeplessness, head heaviness, indigestion, chronic constipation, bone pain, body pain, heart issues, mental weakness, and depression.

- Hair turns gray early, dizziness, and a feeling of helplessness.

- People addicted to self-pleasure lose the ability to think about anything more important, hindering self-awareness.

- The joy from self-pleasure lasts seconds, while the resulting sadness and lack of interest stick around for days.

- Tiredness sets in quickly after self-pleasure, draining a lot of energy.

- Loss of calcium and excess seminal fluid contribute to lower back pain.

- Too much self-pleasure leads to memory loss, as the chemicals in semen are crucial for brain function.

- Work gets disrupted due to addiction and strong sexual urges.

- Hours spent on watching explicit content result in a loss of time, sleep, and energy.

- Excessive sexual thoughts lead to an unsteady mind, disrupting mental stability and focus.

- Experiencing a lot of wet dreams during sleep.

- Hair loss happens due to excessive self-pleasure, affecting DHT levels and preventing hair growth.

- Too much self-pleasure makes you feel intoxicated, like with alcohol and tobacco.

- Excessive loss of vital fluids speeds up the aging process.

- Too much self-pleasure leads to a decrease in sperm count

- Mental imbalance and excessive depression may lead to thoughts of suicide. Feelings of Insecurity and Loneliness

- People may feel deeply insecure and lonely, lacking guidance toward real life satisfaction.

- Ignoring personal experiences is the most harmful effect of too much self-pleasure, as true knowledge comes from your own experiences.

This section is a clear reminder of the many problems caused by excessive masturbation, encouraging readers to think about their own experiences and find a path to true happiness beyond just physical pleasure.

The Hidden Risks of Masturbation

In an article for Psychology Today, Michael Shelton discusses some serious questions about masturbation in sex education for young adults and sometimes parents. He points out that while masturbation is generally considered a healthy and normal behavior, it can occasionally lead to harm. Shelton mentions cases where excessive masturbation caused discomfort, and individuals faced issues like getting caught or stuck while attempting unconventional methods. Despite these instances, masturbation is generally seen as a healthy behavior for guys. However, Shelton emphasizes its role in the development and maintenance of paraphilias. Paraphilias are defined by the American Psychiatric Association as recurring, intense sexual fantasies, urges, or behaviors causing distress or impairment in various aspects of life. Some well-known paraphilias include:

- Pedophilia: Sexual activity with a prepubescent child

- Exhibitionism: Exposing genitals to an unsuspecting stranger

- Frotteurism: Touching and rubbing against a nonconsenting person

- Transvestic fetishism: Sexual arousal to cross-dressing

There are lesser-known paraphilias that still significantly impact many males, such as coprophilia, necrophilia, klismaphilia, and asphyxiophilia. Despite the challenges, most men with socially or legally problematic paraphilias attempt to hide their arousal patterns and engage in more traditional sexual activities.

Addressing the issue, Shelton highlights the reluctance of individuals to disclose their paraphilic attractions, leading to potential negative consequences. He notes that paraphilias have been overlooked in psychology and sex therapy due to the lack of prevalence and treatment outcome studies and the hidden nature of these conditions. Despite potential negative impacts like shame, guilt, and depression, studying paraphilias poses challenges, including dishonesty in self-reporting and the ethical issues of experimental studies. Moreover, the statistical rarity of paraphilia makes longitudinal studies of child and adolescent sexual development less informative.[51]

Navigating Masturbation's Impact with the RECLAiM Team

The Reclaim team, part of Elizabeth Ministry International, comprises experts who hold a distinctive view on masturbation addiction.

While our culture often portrays masturbation as a "healthy release," the Reclaim team aligns with the Catholic Church's teaching that considers masturbation inappropriate. If you're grappling with breaking the habit, you're aware of the detrimental impact it can have on your life. People worldwide approach the RECLAiM team with various questions as they navigate the negative effects of masturbation.

Common queries include:

- "Is there an acceptable amount of masturbation?"

- "If I refrain from masturbation, what alternatives are there for relief?"

- "Can masturbation be a suitable alternative if my spouse cannot or won't engage in sex?"

Recent research in brain science provides fresh insights into this intricate topic. From a neurological standpoint, masturbation is essentially "self-sex," presenting three challenges:[52]

1. The neurochemical rush from sexual experiences can transform masturbation into a convenient escape or self-medication, creating a chemical dependency or addiction over time.

2. Masturbation can disrupt healthy marital sexuality. Neurochemicals that enhance spousal intimacy redirect desire toward oneself rather than one's spouse, making "self-sex" the brain's preferred method for sexual gratification.

3. Masturbation contradicts God's plan for sexuality, meant to be self-giving with love. Acting on lust for self-gratification cheats both the individual and the spouse of the powerful potential inherent in human sexuality. Habitual masturbation may lead to a selfish and lustful perspective on life.

Role of Sex From Progeny to Having Fun

Sex has been super important in how life has evolved on Earth. It's the main way living things make more of themselves. In the animal world, sex happens at specific times, all about making babies, and animals don't overthink it like humans do. But let's look at humans – something interesting is going on. Making babies is still important, but our approach to sex is way more than just reproduction. This section explores how sex has shifted from its basic purpose to becoming a fun and enjoyable part of human culture.

So, in animals, the big deal about sex is making new life. It's a natural thing, timed for survival. Now, think about humans – we've taken sex to a whole new level. It's not just about making babies anymore. We have sex whenever we want, not just when nature says so. We've kind of separated the act from its original purpose. Nowadays, you can't ignore the fact that our culture is flooded with sexual images, and there's this idea that having an active sex life is key to being happy. It's like sex has become as important as other big things we chase after, like money, power, and status.

In our world today, the main idea has shifted from being disciplined about things to just indulging in whatever makes us happy. The message is clear: having a lively sex life is a must for good health and happiness. But stepping away from the original purpose of sex towards a more playful approach makes us wonder – what does this mean for us as individuals and for society as a whole? Comparing the original purpose of sex with how we see it now, filled with pleasure, makes us think about the big cultural influences at work.

It's not a coincidence that humans deal with various sexual and degenerative illnesses that animals don't experience. According to H.P. Blavatsky, when people started treating the sacred act of procreation as mere animal pleasure, we ended up as vulnerable beings. We inherited a range of health issues, making us the most aware but also the most beastly creatures on Earth.[53]

CHAPTER XIII

Distressing Facts of Sexual Health

Every day, over 1 million people worldwide contract sexually transmitted diseases (STDs). Annually, there are 131 million new cases of chlamydia, 78 million of gonorrhea, 5.6 million of syphilis, and 143 million of trichomonas. At any given time, more than 500 million individuals are dealing with genital herpes, and over 290 million women have a human papilloma virus (HPV) infection. Complications like fetal and neonatal deaths, as well as increased risks for infants, are associated with syphilis during pregnancy. HPV infection leads to 528,000 cases of cervical cancer and 266,000 cervical cancer deaths each year. The growing prevalence of oral sex is linked to an increase in throat and mouth cancer due to HPV transmission. Gonorrhea and chlamydia contribute significantly to pelvic inflammatory disease and infertility in women. Additionally, STDs are becoming more resistant to antibiotics, limiting treatment options.[54]

STDs in the United States

In the United States, 1 in 4 teenagers gets an STD annually, and by age 25, half of sexually active young adults will have an STD. Genital herpes affects 45 million people aged 12 and older, marking a 30% increase since the late 1970s.[55] Over 81% of syphilis cases in the U.S. are among gay and bisexual men, who are 17 times more likely to get anal cancer than heterosexual men.[56] Similar trends are observed in England, where gay or bisexual men represent a significant portion of syphilis, gonorrhea, and chlamydia diagnoses.[57]

Contraception and Unintended Pregnancies

Despite efforts to avoid unintended pregnancies, approximately 40% of all pregnancies are unplanned. The contraceptive pill, used by over 100 million people globally, aims to prevent fertilization by altering the female reproductive system. However, it comes with side effects ranging from headaches and irregular bleeding to more severe issues like high blood pressure, liver tumors, and blood clots.[58]

Global Impact of Abortions

Globally, over 55 million abortions occur each year, with nearly half considered unsafe, especially in developing countries with restrictive abortion laws.[59] Approximately 68,000 women die annually due to unsafe abortions, and millions suffer complications, both physical and emotional.[60] Even "safe" procedures can lead to a range of physical side effects, and emotional consequences like guilt, shame, and depression are common.[61]

Internet Pornography and Addiction

About 10% of internet users admit to being addicted to pornography, with 4.2 million pornographic websites and 68 million daily pornographic search engine requests. The average age of first exposure to internet pornography is 11 years, and 34% of internet users experience unwanted exposure to sexual material.[62] Internet pornography addiction has documented negative effects,[63] leading to a growing online community focused on breaking the habit.[64]

Complexities of Sexual Satisfaction

Sexual arousal puts the body in a stressed state, lowering natural defenses and increasing vulnerability to disease. While orgasm is often interpreted as pleasure, it doesn't bring lasting satisfaction, potentially leading to a cycle of arousal and discharge. Frequent sexual indulgence can turn into addiction, and Eastern traditions view compulsive, recreational sex as a weakness. Physiological effects of sex include increased heart rate, respiratory rate, and blood pressure, with potential consequences like fainting, vomiting, and, in extreme cases, even death.[65]

Emotional and Chemical Consequences

Post-sex, partners may experience emotional alienation and "hangover periods" linked to changes in brain chemistry, including dopamine surges.[66] Levels of oxytocin fall after sex, leading to a sense of sexual satiation. Intense sex can cause irritability, dissatisfaction, anxiety, or depression for up to two weeks. Stressful relationships elevate cortisol levels, negatively impacting health.[67] Despite common perceptions, physical sex doesn't guarantee happiness, with studies suggesting that activities like watching TV, helping others, and pursuing hobbies often bring more pleasure than sex.[68]

Physical sex is often overrated as a source of happiness and love. Many of us have experienced the negative consequences of sex, such as conflicts, misunderstandings, and disappointments. We may not realize that sex is just a physical act that cannot heal our emotional pain or increase our joy and satisfaction. ... I strongly believe that one of the causes of marital unhappiness is the unrealistic expectation that our partner should fulfill us sexually. When this does not happen, or when we fail to reciprocate, we feel hurt, angry, and rejected.[69]

Another reason to practice sexual moderation, especially for males, is the health impact of semen loss. Semen contains various substances that are vital for the body, such as sugars, salts, enzymes, vitamins and minerals, including fructose, sorbitol, inositol, phosphorus, zinc, magnesium, calcium, potassium, ascorbic acid (vitamin C) and cobalamin (vitamin B12).[70] When these substances are depleted, the body suffers from weakness and fatigue, and has to work harder to replenish them. On the other hand, when semen is preserved, it is reabsorbed into the bloodstream and used to nourish the body's tissues, especially the brain and nervous system.

Brain cells and semen have a high similarity in their lecithin, chlolesterin and phosphorus contents. Hinduism teaches that semen is a sacred fluid, a creative force, which enhances physical health, moral strength, intellectual power and spiritual growth when conserved. This view was shared by the French writer Honoré de Balzac, who, after a night of passion, would regret: 'There goes another novel!' Athletes and prize fighters are often advised to abstain from sex before a big event, and according to ancient wisdom it is beneficial to avoid sex before any major physical or mental challenge.

Conserving semen is highlighted in Hinduism as a sacred and creative force contributing to physical health, moral stamina, intellectual vigor, and spiritual growth. Loss of semen is associated with a devitalizing effect on the body. Additionally, foreign sperm is proposed as a potential major cause of cancers and other diseases. Sperm, when introduced into another person's body, can lead to various health issues, and the conservation of one's own sperm is advocated for its potential health benefits.[71]

In conclusion, sexual health encompasses a broad range of physical, emotional, and societal aspects, and understanding these complexities is essential for informed decision-making and overall well-being.

The Other Guy's Sperm: The Cause of Cancers and Other Diseases by Donald E. Tyler, M.D. presents a theory that diseases are caused by sperm from other men. Sperm can enter the body by eating or anal sex, which is like cannibalism or organ transplants. Sperm can also invade the tissues and blood vessels of the genitals and spread to other organs. Sperm have a powerful ability to divide and produce any kind of cell, which can lead to cancer and other abnormal growths. Sperm can also trigger immune reactions that attack the body's own cells and organs, causing diseases like arthritis, diabetes, and lupus.

The author presented evidence from experiments, clinics, and studies to support his theory and discussed how sperm are involved in AIDS, urinary infections, birth defects, heart disease, and animal sex. The main idea is that diseases are caused by foreign sperm, either from other men or from the same man in a woman. Sperm from other men can get into the penis of a later sex partner from the vagina of a woman who had sex with them. Foreign sperm are the key factor in diseases. They are probably the main cause of cancers and many other serious diseases.

Donald E. Tyler, M.D. writes, many human diseases remain mysterious, despite extensive research on microbes, parasites, and their effects on the host. For instance, the causes of the common cold, rheumatic fever, eye inflammation, stomach and intestinal ulcers, kidney inflammation, bladder inflammation, endometriosis, rheumatoid arthritis, lupus, dermatomyositis, psoriasis, brain disorders, multiple sclerosis, amyotrophic lateral sclerosis, diabetes, atherosclerosis, birth defects, and tumors are still unknown or unproven. Even for inherited diseases, the origin of gene mutations is unclear. Sperm can penetrate the sensitive tissues of the male and female genitals. Often, there is no visible sign or symptom of infection at the entry point.

Sometimes, there are infections that cause pus and mucus to come out of the male urethra, which are diagnosed as gonorrhea or urethritis. Sperm may also cause ulcers or sores on the genitals that resemble the mouth sores. These ulcers are usually diagnosed as herpes, chanchroid, or syphilis. After entering the genitals, sperm can get into the bloodstream. Sperm or their components can cause lesions throughout the body, which are the root cause of most cancers and adult diseases. The scientific evidence is clear. Sperm are invasive and can enter tissues and cells.

They contain DNA and RNA, which are similar to the genetic material of bacteria and viruses that cause diseases. They are also highly antigenic, which means they trigger an immune response and antibody production. These antigens can also cause inflammation and other reactions. Sperm have all the necessary factors to cause inflammation, and this is observed when sperm leak into the tissues after a vasectomy. When sperm or their parts get into tissues or cells, they may not remain as whole sperm, but may break up into smaller pieces. These pieces can survive, multiply, and behave like they do after fertilization.

When a sperm enters a cell, it can result in a pregnancy-like situation, where new types of cells, including cancers, can grow. Sperm can also cause inflammation to try to eliminate or neutralize them. DNA or its parts, including genes, can be transferred by sperm, as shown by laboratory and clinical experiments. There is evidence that sperm can commonly transfer DNA or its parts. This can lead to diseases that are associated with abnormal chromosomes, genes, and DNA. When sperm or their parts get into the body, they are like a cell transplant; and cells that result from the fusion of sperm or their parts with host cells are another type of cell transplant. The body may try to reject either or both types of transplants, either quickly or slowly, or not at all. The signs of disease may not be noticeable, or they may be mild or severe.

The prostate is a gland the size of a walnut that is located between the bladder and rectum, and makes some of the fluid in semen. 15% of men have prostate inflammation (prostatitis) at some time in their lives; the cause may be bacterial or non-bacterial.[72] when a man gets sexually aroused, all the pelvic reproductive organs, including the prostate, fill up with blood. John Tilden, MD claimed that when the prostate is constantly exposed to this swelling, it gets inflamed and enlarged; this can block the flow of urine, and the prostate may finally turn into a fibrous tumour.[73]

Prostate cancer is the most prevalent cancer among men in the western world, and the second leading cause of cancer death in men after lung cancer. The risk of getting prostate cancer depends on age, genetics, diet, lifestyle, medications and other factors. Many studies have shown that sexually transmitted infections (especially gonorrhea and syphilis), having a lot of sexual partners, or being very sexually active can raise prostate cancer risk by up to 40%.[74]

Other factors that increase cancer risk include being overweight and eating animal fats (especially red meat). A few studies have found a link between high ejaculation frequency and lower prostate cancer risk. A study by Giles et al. (2003) caused misleading media headlines around the world (and all over the internet) that masturbation protects against prostate cancer – but Giles' inconclusive study did not collect any data on masturbation at all.[75]

For women, it is widely believed that they cannot avoid losing mucus and blood during premenstrual and menstrual periods, along with vital substances such as iodine, lecithin, calcium, phosphorus, iron and sex hormones.

The truth is that ovulation does not have to be followed by often painful and long-lasting menstruation; bleeding or breaking of blood vessels is not natural or normal.[76] Leucorrhoea and heavy menstrual bleeding are caused by an inflammation of the lining of the uterus. Frequent sex (especially if it starts at a young age) can also cause chronic inflammation of the vagina and uterus, as well as other genital problems, which can sometimes become cancerous, such as cervical cancer. Wild animals, except for some apes, go through regular cycles of 'heat' without any noticeable blood loss, while domesticated animals do menstruate, because of being confined, overfed and sexually overactive. It is also important to note that women bleed much more heavily in 'civilized' societies than in 'primitive' societies, and prostitutes more so than nuns, for example.

Evidence suggests that excessive sexual behaviour (and erotic fantasies) and a high-protein meat diet are important factors in menstruation, and many women have reduced or stopped menstruation by adopting a healthier diet and lifestyle. Diet has a big impact on sexual desire and behaviour. Meat, fish, shellfish, eggs, salt, spices, onions, garlic, alcohol, (nonherbal) tea, coffee and tobacco, for example, can all act as aphrodisiacs. Animal products, especially meat and seafood, contain uric acid, which irritates and inflames the genital tissues, causing sexual arousal. A low-protein vegetarian diet, on the other hand, tends to have the opposite effect.[77] Overeating is common in the wealthy North, and is linked to the high rates of obesity, cardiovascular diseases and diabetes. In a wartime experiment, 32 men lowered their food intake from 1700 to 1400 calories daily for six months. They reported that sexual desire, erotic dreams, nocturnal ejaculations and aggressive impulses almost vanished.[78]

Dr Edwin Flatto compares the effects of sex and exercise on the body and writes: Sex is mainly catabolic (destructive metabolic action). Sexual arousal makes the blood pile up in the pelvic and reproductive organs of the body. Sexual intercourse involves the loss of vital fluids that have the most important elements and hormones. Sex weakens the person and puts a strain on the heart. Exercise is anabolic (constructive metabolic action). It involves physical activity that develops and keeps physical fitness. It is necessary movement for making the muscles strong and healthy. Proper exercise helps and strengthens all the vital organs, improves the blood flow, and strengthens the heart muscles.[79]

In the plant kingdom, after a plant produces fruit it weakens and often dies. Annuals that flower when only a few weeks old die in a few months. Apple and orange trees live much longer than peach trees, because they grow more slowly and produce fruit later. Nut trees produce fruit even later in life and many live more than 1000 years. By cutting off buds to stop flowering and seeding, the life of the plant is extended, and annuals may become biennials or perennials.

In the animal kingdom, too, reproduction is essentially a movement towards death. The Pacific salmon, trout, shad, and several other types of anadromous fish die soon after spawning. Male drone bees and male spiders usually die soon after, or even during, mating; the male of the black widow spider is sometimes so weak afterwards that the female eats him. Higher animals are much less likely to die after sex but, as a general rule, the earlier an animal reaches puberty and the more often it mates, the shorter its lifespan.[80]

A study of male crickets found that, when they lived with sexually mature females that could reproduce, they were more likely to make high-quality sperm than when they lived with females that could not reproduce, and that making high-quality sperm had a bad effect on their immune systems.[81] In the human kingdom, spiritual mastery and the development of the highest occult powers need perfect self-control and are not compatible with sexual indulgence.[82] By living lives of extreme purity, mahatmas are said to be able to live in the same body for several hundred years if they want.[83] Among other things, sex has bad effects on the 'third eye', the organ of spiritual vision.

Theosophy says that in the third root-race this was a real physiological organ located at the back of the head, but as evolution went down the 'arc of descent' (into matter), and spirituality was replaced by 'the newly-awakened physiological and psychic passions of the physical man', it gradually lost its powers and shrivelled.[84]

The pineal gland is an endocrine gland that looks like a pine cone and is located in the middle of the brain within the third cerebral ventricle. The pineal is our main gland; it turns light, temperature and magnetic information from our surroundings into neuroendocrine signals that control the body's functioning. In some lower vertebrates the pineal gland has a well-formed eye-like structure, while in others it acts as a light sensor. This pineal, or parietal, eye is now widely seen by science as the evolutionary ancestor of the modern eye.

The powerful Hindu God Shiva is called 'the great ascetic' and is revered as an example of celibacy and ascetic power. His third eye is said to be the outcome of his perfect purity.

The pineal gland makes the hormone melatonin, which affects sleeping cycles, biorhythms and sexual development. It is big in children and starts to shrink with the start of puberty. Lecithin, an organic phosphorized fat, is a main component not only of semen but also of brain and nerve tissue, and the pineal gland has more lecithin than any other part of the body. During sexual arousal, impulses are sent up the spinal cord to the brain, and this stops the 'reopening' of the spiritual eye. It is said that in the seventh root-race, millions of years from now, the pineal gland will once again become active in all humans as the organ for the seventh sense – spiritual intuition.[85]

Semen and Time: Accepting the Unrecoverable Loss

Swami Shivananda, a famous spiritual guru in his *"The Practice of Brahmacharya"* writes, the sex pleasure is the most weakening and depressing of pleasures. Sensual enjoyment comes with various faults. It comes with various kinds of sins, pains, weaknesses, attachments, slave mentality, weak will, hard work and struggle, craving and mental restlessness. Worldly people never regain their proper senses even though they get harsh hits, kicks and blows from different sides. The wandering street dog never stops from going to the houses even though it is thrown with stones every time. Famous doctors of the West say that various kinds of diseases come from the loss of semen, especially in young age. There appear boils on the body, acne or eruptions on the face, blue lines around the eyes, lack of beard, sunken eyes, pale face with anemia, loss of memory, loss of eye-sight, shortsightedness, discharge of semen along with urine, enlargement of the testes, pain in the testes, weakness, sleepiness, laziness, gloominess, palpitation of the heart, dyspnoea or trouble in breathing, phthisis, pain in the back, loins, head and joints, weak kidneys, passing urine in sleep, fickle-mindedness, lack of thinking power, bad dreams, wet dreams and restlessness of mind. Notice carefully the evil after-effects that follow the loss of seminal energy! People are physically, mentally and morally weakened by wasting the seminal power on so many occasions for nothing. The body and the mind refuse to work strongly. There is physical and mental tiredness.

You experience much exhaustion and weakness. You will have to resort to drinking milk, to eating fruits and aphrodisiac confections, to make up for the loss of energy. Remember that these things can never, never repair the loss fully. Once lost is lost forever. You will have to live a dull, joyless existence. Bodily and mental strength gets reduced day by day. Those who have lost much of their Veerya become very irritable. Little things disturb their minds. Those who have not followed the vow of celibacy become the slaves of anger, jealousy, laziness and fear. If you have not got your senses under control, you risk to do foolish acts which even children will not do.

He who has wasted the vital energy becomes easily irritable, loses his balance of mind and gets into a state of explosive fury for trivial things. When a man becomes furious, he behaves badly. He does not know what he is exactly doing as he loses his power of reasoning and discrimination. He will do anything he likes. He will insult even his parents, Guru and respectable people. It is important, therefore, that the aspirant who is trying to develop good behaviour must preserve the vital energy. Preservation of this divine energy leads to the attainment of strong will-power, good behaviour, spiritual elevation, and Sreyas or Moksha eventually. Too much sexual intercourse drains the energy greatly. Young men do not understand the value of the vital fluid. They waste this dynamic energy by excessive copulation. Their nerves are stimulated much. They become drunk.

What a serious mistake they make! It is a crime that deserves capital punishment. They are killers of Atman. When this energy is once wasted, it can never be regained by any other means. It is the most powerful energy in the world. One sexual act breaks completely the brain and the nervous system. People foolishly think that they can recover the lost energy by taking milk, almonds and Makaradhvaja. This is a mistake. You must try your best to preserve every drop even though you are a married man. Self-realization is the goal.

The energy that is lost during one sexual intercourse is equal to the energy that is used in physical work for ten days or the energy that is needed for mental work for three days. Notice how valuable is the vital fluid, semen! Do not lose this energy. Keep it with great care. You will have amazing vitality. When semen is not wasted, it is all changed into Ojas Sakti or spiritual energy and kept in the brain. Western doctors know little of this important point. Most of your diseases are due to too much seminal loss.[86]

Nature's Influence: Understanding Involuntary Semen Release

Swami Shivananda on wet dreams said wet dream and voluntary copulation—a vital difference. A sexual act breaks the nervous system. The whole nervous system is disturbed or agitated during the act. There is a lot of loss of energy. More energy is lost during coition. But it is not the same when emission happens during the dreaming state. In a wet dream, it may be the outflow of the prostatic fluid only. Even if there is loss of the vital fluid, there is not much draining. The actual essence does not come out during wet dreams. It is only the watery prostatic fluid with a little semen that is released during nocturnal pollutions.

When nocturnal emission happens, the mind which was working in the inner astral body suddenly enters the physical body strongly in an agitated state. That is the reason why emission happens suddenly. The night discharge may not arouse the sexual desire. But a voluntary copulation, in the case of a sincere aspirant is very harmful to his spiritual progress.

The Samskara created by the act will be very deep; and it will increase or strengthen the force of the previous Samskaras that are already in the subconscious mind and will arouse the sexual desire. It will be like pouring ghee in the fire that is slowly dying out. The task of removing this new Samskara will be a hard work. You should totally give up copulation. This mind will try to deceive you in many ways by giving wrong advice. Be on the alert. Do not listen to its voice, but try to listen to the voice of the conscience or the voice of the soul or the voice of discrimination. Nocturnal discharge, night pollution, Svapna-Dosha, wet dream are all the same terms.

Ayurvedic doctors call this disease Sukra Megha. This is due to the bad habits in youth. In severe cases, discharges happen in daytime also. The patient passes semen along with urine during urination. If there is occasional discharge, you need not be worried a bit. This may be due to heat in the body, or the pressure of full bowels or bladder on the seminal bags. This is not a pathological condition. Night pollution is of two kinds, namely, physiological pollution and pathological pollution. In physiological pollution, you will be refreshed.

You should not be scared of this act. You should not care if the discharge of semen is very occasional. You need not worry about it. This is also a slight cleaning of the apparatus or a periodic cleansing through a slight overflow from the reservoir in which the semen is kept up. This act may not be attended with evil thoughts. The person may not be aware of the act during the night. Whereas, in pathological pollution, the act is accompanied by sexual thoughts and depression follows. There is irritability, weakness, laziness, inability to work and focus. Occasional discharges are of no importance, but frequent nocturnal pollutions cause low mood, weakness, indigestion, low spirits, loss of memory, severe pain in the back, headache, burning of the eyes, sleepiness and burning sensation at urination or during the flow of semen. The semen becomes very thin.[87]

A man who keeps the seminal fluid for twelve years gains a special power. He develops a new inner nerve called the nerve of memory. Through that nerve he recalls all, he comprehends all. Loss of semen weakens the strength. But it does not harm one if one loses it in a dream. That semen one gets from food. What stays after nocturnal discharge is enough. The semen that stays after nocturnal discharge is very 'pure'. The Lahas stored jars of molasses in their house. Every jar had a hole in it. After a year they found that the molasses had hardened like sugar candy. The extra watery part had dripped out through the hole.[88]

A common misconception is that men need to ejaculate regularly, otherwise they will have wet dreams. This is false, because unused semen does not build up in the body, but is absorbed back into the blood. There is no proof that men who abstain from sex have more wet dreams than men who have sex. Wet dreams are usually caused by irritation and swelling of the urinary tube, due to too much sexual activity and/or spicy food. Other reasons for wet dreams are pressure on the sperm sacs from a bloated (constipated) bowel and a full bladder.[89]

Physiological, Psychological And Social Harms Of Masturbation - Experts' Excerpts

Physical Harms of Masturbation[90]

Undoubtedly, masturbation can cause physical harm, though some may exaggerate its effects. Medical science has confirmed several diseases linked to it, including:

- Weakening of sexual organs and partial looseness.

- General weakening of nerves due to exertion.

- Impact on limb growth, especially the outer part of the urethra.

- Creation of seminal inflammation in the testicles, leading to quick sperm ejaculation.

- Pain in the vertebra column, causing back crookedness and twisting.

- Shaking and shivering in limbs like the legs.

- Weakness in cerebral glands affecting perception, reasoning, and memory.

- Weakening of eyesight, reducing normal vision limits.

- Premature aging effects.

- Weakening of delicate nerves and veins, causing sexual impotency.

- Excessive sperm loss through nocturnal emission (wet dreams).

- Decrease in the body's natural resistance.

- Harm to vital organs: heart, brain, liver, and stomach.

- Reduction in natural animal heat, vital for soul and body strength.

- Excessive loss of blood due to sperm production.

- Weakening of the bladder.

Psychological and Social Harms

- Psychologists note an internal struggle in youth practicing this act, feeling aware of wrongdoing and sin.

- Excessive practice leads to cowardice, increased nervous agitation, lack of self-confidence, disgrace, reduced study urge, and a tendency towards isolation.

- Addiction and attachment may develop, diverting from using it to satisfy desires to practicing it compulsively.

CHAPTER XIV

The Anatomy of Crimes of Sexual Desire

What drives people to commit crimes? What makes them cross the line between morality and immorality, between law and lawlessness, between right and wrong? There are many possible answers to these questions, but one of the most common and powerful factors is sexual desire.

Sexual desire, or lust, is a natural and universal human instinct. It is the source of life, love, and pleasure. But it can also be the source of death, hate, and pain. When sexual desire is misdirected, abused, or overstimulated, it can lead to a variety of crimes, both sexual and non-sexual, that harm individuals and society.

C. J. VanVliet, in his book *The Coil Serpent* has evidently argued sexual immorality and perversion are the main causes of many crimes, and that people who indulge in lustful thoughts and emotions are partly responsible for the crimes committed by others. The society can definitely get a good lesson that reducing sexual desire and restoring its natural function would lead to less crime and more happiness.

Many crimes are motivated by sexual passion, which draws the attention of both moralists and judges, as well as the many victims who suffer from it. Sexual crimes are among the most tragic aspects of modern criminality, and they are evident in many cases of murder, jealousy, and deviance. Moreover, the unnatural sexual relations that characterize our artificial civilization are the source of the widespread vice and crime in our times.

It is not surprising that crime is increasing, since most of the sexual acts of humanity are unnatural and corrupt. Sex acts as a trigger for crime, just as alcohol acts as a trigger for sexual interest.

When sexual lust is unleashed, it ignites all kinds of wickedness. There is no evil intention or action that sexual pleasure will not make a person do. This is especially clear in the delinquency of young people, who often start their criminal career with illicit sexual indulgence. Experts have also observed that young criminals tend to be sexually precocious.

This supports the view of philosophers who have claimed that sexual excitement is the greatest evil of all, and that lust is the root of all evil. The way humanity has misused and overstimulated the sexual urge is the main reason for most of the misery that afflicts mankind.

If lust were limited to its natural purpose of preserving the race, there would be much less crime, since the biggest temptation would be removed. Therefore, it is urgent that law enforcement pays more attention to the close connection between sex and crime. Of course, most people think that they are far from committing or being involved in any crime. However, few are completely innocent of sharing the guilt of those who commit sexual crimes. Some of the guilt falls on those who entertain erotic thoughts and feelings.

It is a common saying that thoughts are things, but few people take seriously the idea that passionate emotions also create various kinds of thought-forms. It seems logical that every small thought or emotion produces a vibratory wave that connects with others of the same nature.

They reinforce each other until they form powerful blocks of emotion-forms that float around and can easily influence people. It seems literally true that sensuality covers humanity with a heavy and gloomy veil, which is always ready to attack the unsuspecting and inject its poison into their emotional system. All who are receptive to it - the young, the weak, the sensual, the criminal - are dangerously exposed to the influence of the terrible thought-forms that many self-righteous people have contributed to. In essence, even the slightest erotic thinking can lead to someone's criminal behavior - which makes the thinker of sensual thoughts a promoter of crime. Considering this, one may conclude that, from a moral point of view, indulging in sexual sensuality is one of the greatest crimes.

To understand it better, let's take an example of the current analysis of Juvenile Justice Bulletin published on December 2009.[91]

The number of young people involved in sexual offenses has increased recently, and there are now specialized treatment and management programs for them. However, we have limited information about the characteristics of these offenders and their offenses on a larger scale. The National Incident-Based Reporting System (NIBRS) sheds light on the characteristics of juvenile sex offenders known to law enforcement. Here are some key findings:

- About 35.[6] percent of those known to police for committing sex offenses against minors are juveniles.

- Juveniles who commit sex offenses against other children are more likely to offend in groups and at schools, with more male and younger victims compared to adult sex offenders.

- The number of youth involved in sex offenses sharply increases at age 12, reaching a plateau after age 14. Early adolescence is the peak age for offenses against younger children, while offenses against teenagers increase during mid to late adolescence.

- A small number of juvenile offenders (1 out of 8) are younger than 12.

- Females make up 7 percent of juvenile sex offenders and are more common among younger offenders. Their offenses often involve multiple victims and perpetrators, and victims may be family members or males.

- Different jurisdictions vary significantly in their concentration of reported juvenile sex offenders.

Research on juvenile sex offenders has been ongoing for over 50 years, with increased interest since the mid-1980s. Treatment programs for juvenile sex offenders have grown, leading to a surge in research articles. Most studies focus on clinical characteristics, treatment issues, risk predictors, and recidivism rates. There is a diversity of behaviors, backgrounds, and motivations among juvenile sex offenders.

Juvenile sex offenders make up more than one-quarter (25.8 percent) of all sex offenders and over one-third (35.6 percent) of sex offenders against juvenile victims. They account for 3.1 percent of all juvenile offenders and 7.4 percent of violent juvenile offenders. About 89,000 juvenile sex offenders were known to police in the United States in 2004. Their ages vary, with the majority being male. Juvenile sex offenders differ from adult sex offenders in various dimensions, including offending in groups, targeting acquaintances, and committing offenses at different locations and times.

The relationship between offender age and victim age varies, and the issue of juvenile sex offenses against minors continues to be a subject of controversy and debate. The NIBRS dataset is a valuable resource for understanding and analyzing this complex problem.

CHAPTER XV

Unseen Impact of Sexual Abuse

I am going to explore how sexual abuse can hurt us in ways we might not even realize. Once again, we'll look at how it affects our bodies, our minds, and even our feelings of love and desire. I am inspired by renowned authors like Torkom Saraydarian and Dr. Edwin Flatto on this most astounding topic.

Think of it as shining a light into the dark corners of a room. We want to bring these hidden effects out into the open so we can understand them better. By doing that, we hope to start a journey toward healing and understanding.

Effects of Sexual Abuse on the Physical Body[92]

1. Sexual abuse weakens your body's defense against diseases, making your immune system less effective. To boost it, take a break from sex when you feel you're absorbing germs.

2. Excessive sexual activity can make your nervous system shaky. Test this by checking if your fingers tremble or if you can stand on one foot without any wobbling.

3. Sexual abuse can lead to laziness and sleepiness. Abstaining for a few months can often bring back enthusiasm, making it easier to wake up early and stay active.

4. Sexual abuse affects the body's color, voice, and energy. Singers, especially, notice the impact. Moderation is crucial for maintaining a great voice.

5. Engaging in sex too early may lead to impotency. Controlling and sublimating the sex drive is essential for sustaining energy, as exemplified by a Russian ballet dancer who limited intimacy to maintain his dancing prowess.

6. Sexual abuse weakens relationships as it drains the vital energy needed to sustain them. Couples who conserve sexual energy often have longer-lasting connections.

7. Abusing sex may result in weak or early-inclined offspring. The energy you carry influences your children, impacting their tendencies.

8. Sexual abuse contributes to various health problems, potentially shortening one's lifespan by several decades.

9. Abusing sexual energy during growth periods may prevent reaching full height. This is particularly concerning for young individuals who might stop growing prematurely.

10. Sexual abuse can weaken eyesight over time.

11. The heart may weaken, leading to potential heart diseases due to sexual abuse.

12. There's a potential link between sexual abuse and cancer development, as the body works overtime to replace drained energy.

13. Sexual abuse may contribute to various organic difficulties within the body.

14. Those who abuse their sexual energy tend to live significantly shorter lives than they otherwise would.

15. Sexual abuse can damage the pineal, pituitary, and carotid glands.

Emotional Effects of Sexual Abuse

1. Nervousness

2. Gossiping Urges

3. Nosiness

4. Irritability

5. Destructiveness

6. Indifference to Responsibilities

7. Inclination Towards Crime

8. Jealousy

9. Selfishness

10. Pessimism

11. Sense of Isolation

12. Hatred for Others' Beauty

13. Sneakiness

14. Loss of Aura Magnetis

Mental Effects of Sexual Abuse

1. Loss of Moral Principles

2. Lack of Achievement Drive

3. Absence of Striving for Knowledge, Service, and Leadership

4. Mental Diffusion

5. Lack of Higher Goals

6. No Contact with Inner Guide

7. Attempting to Exploit Others

8. Misleading Behavior

9. Development of Hatred and Separatism

10. Lying

11. Vanity

12. Showcasing

13. Various Complicated Mental Problems and Insanity

Spiritual Effects of Sexual Abuse

1. Hindered Connection to Higher Spiritual Energies

2. Loss of Energy in Knowledge Petals, Resulting in Confusion

3. Potential Obsession

4. Damaged Throat Center

5. Decreased Creative Energy in the Mental Body

6.   Ugly Imagination Development

7.   Polluted Aura Hindering Contact with Forces of Nature

8.   Disruption of Telepathic Communication

9.   Increased Karma

10. Complicated Relationships

11. Detrimental Impact on Children's Future

I don't care if sex is bad for my health[93]

Some people might respond to this book by saying, "I don't care if sex is bad for my health, I don't want to hear about it!" But I firmly believe that information is always beneficial. When a person knows the facts, he can make smart choice. Let's begin with the assumption that sex is a vital function. Is this true? Physically, sex is not the same as other natural, normal, bodily functions like eating, breathing, sleeping, defecating, or urinating.

We need to do these things regularly and constantly to survive. But many healthy people have shown that a person can live a long and healthy life without ever having sex. The idea of necessity is based on preference. In fact, there is no disease caused by not having sex, but there are many diseases caused by having too much sex. This book does not promote total abstinence or celibacy as a lifestyle. I just want to make clear at the start that there is nothing wrong with being chaste. Sex is not a vital function that has to be done frequently. The organs and glands that control reproduction are not like our muscles that need to be exercised frequently to work well. Actually, the opposite is true: the reproductive glands work better and stronger when they have a break. The assumption that sex is natural also needs to be challenged. It depends on how it is used.

Nature clearly designed the sexual organs for reproduction, not for fun. If our Creator wanted us to have sex for pleasure only, there would be no need for all the effort, time, and huge amounts of money spent on finding a safe and effective birth control method without negative or unwanted side effects. Man is the only animal that nature allows, in his natural habitat, to have sex whenever he wants. All the other animals have specific mating seasons when the female will accept the male organ. These are the brief periods when the female can get pregnant, or is in 'rut' or 'heat.' The female dog will not let a male dog have sex with her unless she is in 'heat' which usually happens once every six months. The same pattern is followed throughout the animal kingdom.

Birds usually mate once a year or in the spring. Sheep and goats mate once or twice a year during their mating seasons. Wild pigs mate once a year, and the elephant, in its wild state, mates only once every two years. Reproduction is basically destructive throughout the animal and plant kingdoms. That is, it leads to death. The Pacific salmon, trout, shad, and several other types of fish that swim upstream to spawn die soon after. The male drone bee dies right after mating. Even more striking is the sex life of the praying mantis. In his book, *Love and Will*, Rollo May writes: 'The female eats the male's head as he mates, and his dying spasms join with his mating spasms to make the thrusts stronger. After being fertilized, the female continues to eat him to store up food for the new offspring.' The black widow spider does basically the same thing and gets its name from this behavior.

In the plant kingdom, after a plant produces fruit it weakens and often dies. Farmers often try to stop a plant or tree from 'going to seed' to make it stronger. Most fruit-bearing trees do not make fruit until they are five to ten years old. This lets their biological energy be used for growth and strength rather than reproduction. Many coaches and trainers in sports ban sexual activity before a competition. Boxers stay away from sex during training and before a fight. The human sperm, of course, has all the key ingredients to make another human being when it joins with the egg. It has powers that can produce life. Isn't it logical to save such an important fluid instead of wasting it carelessly? Some people still believe that oysters, steak, liquor, etc., boost sexual performance. Stimulants make the desire stronger but the ability weaker. I think you will agree that it is much better to have less desire and more ability! ... Many men, even after realizing the damage they are causing to themselves by having too much sex, continue with their old habits. They say that they cannot control themselves in sex. I admit that it is hard. But not impossible! It is good for you to do hard things.

Self-discipline is a skill that gets better with practice. It is a mental muscle. I only support moderation. Indulgence lowers a man's noble nature. To claim that humans cannot do what requires self-control is to deny their higher, though maybe hidden, nature. Sensual men, who want to satisfy every craving, will only get what they deserve from nature: painful illness and early death.

Love and Lust: Understanding the Difference

In the wise words of Henry David Thoreau, "Love and lust are as far asunder as a flower garden is from a brothel." This means they're quite different. Love and sex operate on opposing principles – love is personal and uplifting, while sex can be more casual and potentially denigrating. Pure love is noble, while pure sex can be demoralizing. Love is unselfish and spiritual, while sex tends to be more physical and self-seeking. Nature has its say too; the reproductive seed holds vital forces for species propagation. Sex is not entertainment. Wasting this substance for amusement harms our health. Sex, in its essence, is a bit like a "destructive utilization of energy" in males, sacrificing important cells for reproduction. Unfortunately, our society often panders to the sex urge instead of promoting sexual discipline.

Birth control pills have become commonplace, but their consequences are not always considered. Regardless of their safety, the mindset behind their use may lead to problems. It's essential to recognize that nature intended sex for procreation, and ignoring these laws can result in mental and physical bankruptcy. Our society's emphasis on pleasure-seeking over self-discipline calls for a reevaluation of our attitudes towards life and the importance of control and restraint.[94]

The Ripple Effect Of Abortion: Challenging the Double Standard in Sex Ethics

In the realm of sex ethics, a longstanding double standard persists, with men historically adhering to lower or no standards while women were held to higher expectations. The accessibility of low-cost abortions, birth control drugs, and contraceptives has granted women the liberty to engage in sexual relations without the natural consequences of pregnancy, shifting the focus from creating life to seeking pleasure. Rather than urging men to meet higher standards, women, in what they perceive as liberation, have aligned their standards with men.

Despite physical disparities favoring men, evidence suggests that women often exceed men morally. Men's chronic state of sexual readiness contributes to societal issues, as seen in violence and explicit content support predominantly by men. Legal abortions, even under optimal conditions, pose severe risks, both immediate and long-term, impacting a woman's future pregnancies. Beyond physical concerns, the moral and spiritual repercussions of abortion challenge the cultivation of respect for the sacredness of human life, a fundamental aspect of our upward spiritual evolution.[95]

Relationship between Sex and Cardiovascular Health

Understanding how sex affects the heart isn't straightforward. Various studies highlight specific points:[96]

- **Heartbeat Differences:** Men generally have faster heartbeats than women.

- **Intercourse Acceleration:** During intercourse, heart rates can speed up significantly, reaching up to 100 beats in a minute.

- **Heartbeat Variations:** Close to orgasm, abnormal and skipped heartbeats often appear, but they don't show up on subsequent ECG tests during nonsexual exercise.

- **Physiological Changes:** From foreplay onwards, heart rates sporadically increase, blood pressure rises (40 to 80 mm systolic, 20 to 50 mm diastolic on average), and respiratory rates sharply climb. Physiologically, sex and exercise have opposite effects on the body.

When it comes to sex, it's like the body goes through some breaking-down stuff. It makes the blood get stuck in certain body parts, like the pelvis and reproductive organs. Because of this, the body loses important fluids with stuff like hormones and elements it needs. This makes us feel weaker and puts more pressure on our hearts. Now, on the other hand, exercise is like the body building itself up. It helps us get in shape, makes our muscles stronger, gets the blood flowing better, and gives our heart a good workout too. So, even though both sex and exercise can make our hearts beat faster, they affect our bodies in very different ways.

CHAPTER XVI

How Sex Could Impact Longevity Negatively

A Common Belief

These findings challenge a common belief that unlimited use of sexual abilities does not harm the physical health of the person, and that limiting the sexual drive may lead to serious disease. Some recent researchers of the sexual behavior of American men and women argue that even the most extreme excesses have no negative impact on health and energy; their work appears to suggest, or has been made to suggest by critics and commentators, that the restrictive rules of our religious, moral, and legal codes should be loosened because the sexually free society is more healthy and happy than the constrained society. A sadly large number of Americans, especially naive young people, eagerly embrace these ideas and use them as an excuse for sex greed.

It should be obvious that these claims are completely unscientific. Their main arguments have never been verified, while their assumed consequences are sheer nonsense. If one questions what evidence these researchers use to support their claims, one finds very little. In recent works like Dr. Kinsey's books, no proof of the accuracy of his data is given. The authors did not put their interviewees through any rigorous examination, nor did they sample a diverse enough range of people to confirm their findings. In the light of today's medical knowledge, their claims, especially about the supposed safety of over indulgence, are false. The available body of evidence clearly shows that excessive sexual activity, especially when it is illegal, has significantly harmful effects.[97]

Detrimental Effects on Longevity

In contrast to above widespread view, a moderate sexual life or complete abstinence shows none of these effects. This is clearly demonstrated when we compare the lives of Christian saints, the Roman Catholic Popes, and distinguished theologians and clerics, with the libertine lives of many monarchs, heirs, heiresses, and stars of screen and stage. An overwhelming majority of Christian saints were ascetics.

In our study of the lives of 3,090, more than 98 per cent lived between the first and the nineteenth centuries.

According to today's standards of hygiene, a large majority of them lived in physical conditions harmful to both health and longevity. Many engaged in countless fasts. They renounced the fulfillment of their bodies' most pressing needs. Some deliberately inflicted pain on themselves. In sum, the regime imposed by religious, monastic, or eremitic rules, or by themselves, was often harsher than that of galley slaves.

On the other hand, many of the monarchs lived in conditions providing the fullest gratification of bodily needs and desires. They enjoyed the best possible standard of living. Their health was monitored by the leading medical experts. However, in their sexual behavior, many were as licentious and voracious as the most extreme profligates. Now, if the prevalent theory regarding the harmfulness of abstinence and the healthfulness of overindulgence of the sexual urge were true, the monarchs would have enjoyed better health and lived longer than the Christian saints. The facts strongly reject this expectation.

A study of the life span of 332 monarchs (Roman and Byzantine emperors, Turkish sultans, Russian czars, and English, French, Austrian, German, Italian, Spanish, Danish kings, and of 3,090 Christian Catholic saints gives the following data about their age at death. In both groups, those who died by violence are excluded.[98]

Age at death	Monarch Percent	Age at death	Saints Percent
Under 40 years	18.0	Under 40 years	19.0
40 to 59 years	44.8	41 to 60 years	26.6
60 to 79 years	34.2	61 to 80 years	37.4
80 to 99 years	3.0	81 to 100 years	14.4
100 years & above	–	101 years & above	2.6

Considering the family traits shared by saints and monarchs, it's reasonable to think that the sexual habits of monarchs might have influenced their shorter lifespans. Monarchs generally had better living conditions than saints, but their excessive behavior might have counteracted those advantages. On the other hand, the self-discipline of saints might have balanced out their less favorable circumstances.[99]

The argument extends to comparing the lifespan of monarchs with that of Roman Catholic Popes. Despite the demanding nature of their roles, Popes lived longer on average. In a period where the influence of Christendom surpassed secular power, Catholic Popes lived to an average age of 69.8 years, compared to the 53 to 54 years for 332 monarchs. This suggests that the continence of Popes contrasted with the sexual indulgence of many monarchs, contributing to their longer lives.[100]

This trend extends to other historically prominent groups. The chastest groups, including Popes, theologians, monks, hermits, and clerics, exhibit the longest lifespans. Conversely, those with more libertine lifestyles, such as poets, musicians, and painters, tend to have shorter lifespans. Monarchs, in particular, have the shortest lifespan among these groups.[101]

These patterns support the idea that excessive sexual activity negatively impacts the longevity of certain groups, while moderation, as seen in saints, Popes, and dedicated individuals, contributes to longer life. This conclusion gains further support when examining contemporary figures known for their sexual exploits. Despite ideal living conditions and expert healthcare, these individuals experience early declines in vitality and numerous health issues in their prime.[102]

In simple terms, let's talk about the health of people who engage in risky behaviors, especially those with limited money. Sadly, many who are involved in these behaviors end up in trouble, often in the company of criminals. This not only harms their health but can also lead to a shorter life. Some manage to avoid serious consequences, but their lives are still tough, marked by danger, lack of basic needs, and disrespect. They struggle to make a living and maintain a good standing in their community, gradually becoming social outcasts with numerous difficulties. This lifestyle drains their energy, ages them faster, and eventually brings them to an early grave. Engaging excessively in risky behaviors, especially those related to sex, seriously damages an individual's physical well-being.[103]

Contrary to a popular belief that controlling sexual desires can lead to illness, it's largely a misconception. Likewise, thinking that unrestricted sexual activity isn't harmful is also not accurate. Believing in these ideas contributes to an increase in risky behavior and, consequently, negatively affects the vitality and lifespan of those who follow them. Scientific studies, like those mentioned by Jatin

Shankar in his book on *modern biological theories,* shed light on the consequences of such behaviors. For instance, experiments show that removing the ability to reproduce can slow down aging in various organisms. This implies that a longer life often comes at the expense of reduced fertility.

A mental hospital in the 20th century castrated some patients who caused trouble. The aim was to make them calmer, but this cruel act also became a scientific study on how castration affects lifespan. The researchers found that the castrated patients lived longer (James B. Hamilton, 1969), and the younger they were when castrated, the more their life expectancy increased. Some notable features of this study are:[104]

- The castrated and intact patients had the same living conditions, so lifestyle factors did not affect lifespan.

- The castrated patients were similar to the rest of the population in every way except behavior, which led to castration. This means that health was not a factor in choosing who to castrate, and the two groups were comparable. This is rare because nowadays castration is done for medical reasons, and such patients cannot be matched with healthy ones.

- The study involved 297 castrated and 735 intact males, so the sample size was large and the errors were minimized. This graph shows the results of the study more clearly.

- This graph illustrates the results of the study more clearly. You can see that 50% of the castrated males lived until 70, while the intact males reached 50% survival at around 55.

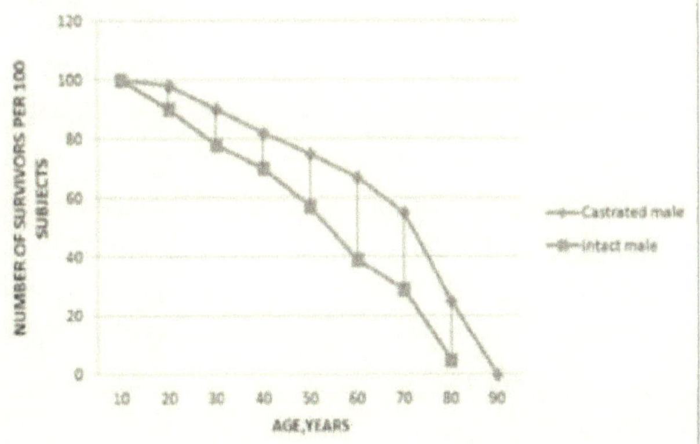

A recent study examined the lifespan of 81 Korean eunuchs from the 16th to 19th centuries based on historical records. The eunuchs lived 14 years longer than the average people at that time, and 3 of them reached over 100 years, indicating slower aging in eunuchs. Eunuchs also had other intriguing features. For example, men who were castrated before or after developing male pattern baldness did not lose or even regained hair (HAMILTON, 1960). These facts suggest that castration has anti-aging effects, which is consistent with previous experiments. Castration also increases the lifespan of other animals like dogs, bulls, mice and salmon (Robertson, 1961). This shows that sexual reproduction, body repair and maintenance have trade-offs with energy allocation and lifespan.[105]

How Sexuality Shaping Society's Downfall

Pitirim Sorokin talks about a strange revolution happening nowadays. It's not about armies or wars, but it involves individuals worldwide. He calls it the 'Sex Revolution,' and it's causing sexual chaos. This revolution is crucial because it greatly affects people and society. In his book, 'Sane Sex Order,' Sorokin discusses how sex chaos harms physical and mental health, creativity, and society. A significant consequence is the breakdown of families, the building blocks of a healthy society.

In the USA and Europe, family life is declining rapidly. In Britain, 150,000 kids under 16 face their parents' divorce each year. Unmarried mothers increased fourfold to 360,000 from 1971-89. In 1980, 12% of births were outside marriage; by 1990, it rose to 28%. Single-parent families now make up 19% of the total, with over 30% of births occurring outside marriage.[106]

In the USA, teenage pregnancy and a doubling divorce rate are major concerns. Two-fifths of kids spend part of their youth in single- parent homes. While children from single-parent families can succeed, on average, they fare worse in various aspects—physically, emotionally, behaviorally, educationally, economically, and even in terms of smoking and drinking. They face earlier mortality, struggle in school, lack proper nourishment, endure higher unemployment, engage in deviance and crime, and are more susceptible to psychiatric illness. The community also suffers, expressing itself through crime, vandalism, and violence. Establishing a sensible sex order and a stable marriage system is crucial sociologically.

Anthropologically, there are various marriage types, like eight described in Hinduism or polygamy in Islam. There are different family structures beyond traditional joint and nuclear families. Even if these traditional forms aren't ideal for industrial societies, the need for care and support from close ones, ideally parents until at least 20, and afterward from a spouse 'in sickness and in health' until death, remains a crucial human aspect.

This need isn't met in a culture dominated by sexual chaos and illicit relationships. Sorokin suggests elevating culture and social life to establish a sane sex order. This involves freeing our culture and institutions from the burden of sexuality. The transformation includes desexualizing fine arts, multimedia, sciences, philosophy, ethics, and law—basically, our entire way of life. Idealizing love, marriage, and family is also part of this significant change. This is the sociological aspect of Brahmacharya, vital even while practicing it in thought, word, and deed.

Sexuality, Creativity, and Cultural Evolution

Let's go further talking about what Pitirim A. Sorokin in the book "*The American Sex Revolution*" says about how sexuality can impact societies. We're asking if disorderly or controlled relationships affect the growth or decline of societies. Does the way people handle their relationships, like being free or more controlled, influence a society's progress or downfall?

A society that limits sex to marriage and disapproves of premarital and extramarital relations is better for creative growth than one where relationships are free-spirited and not regulated. Too much disorderly behavior harms the society's creativity. The evidence for these ideas comes from the negative effects of excessive and illicit sex behavior discussed earlier.

Some real-life examples back this up, like the experiences in Soviet Russia and China, where more sexual freedom led to problems. The book also mentions how different societies with various cultural levels had different views on sex freedom.

Let's look at the history of cultures. Among preliterate societies, those with more prenuptial freedom tended to have a certain mindset. As societies progressed, they tended to restrict premarital and extramarital relations, leading to more creativity. The societies that strictly limited sexual freedom reached higher cultural levels.

For instance, when Christianity influenced the Teutonic tribes, limiting sexual freedom played a vital role in their cultural progress. On the flip side, when societies relaxed their rules, like in later stages of Babylonian, Persian, and Roman civilizations, there was a decline.

Now, let's talk about experiments in Soviet Russia in the 1920s. They initially tried to destroy marriage and promote free love, but it led to issues like homelessness among children. Eventually, they had to change their approach, promoting premarital chastity and the importance of marriage. Similar changes are happening in Communist China now, showing that controlling previously encouraged sex freedom can be beneficial. This idea is backed by examples of colonial peoples facing demoralization due to Western culture's impact.

Contrastingly, among Hindus, Indonesians, and Indo-Chinese, their societies revived under a new gospel of sexual restraint. Leaders like Gandhi supported this idea. Now, let's bring this closer to home - the impact on families. When a family's sexual life becomes disorderly, it can lead to the family breaking down and producing societal issues like mental illness, crime, and addiction.

Moving on to economic development, the book mentions that Europe's economic growth started with groups that practiced sexual restraint. But when ethical standards lowered, especially in terms of sexual freedom, the capitalist system began to decline. Summing it up, too much focus on sexual activities for a prolonged period can drain energy, leaving little for creativity. On the other hand, individuals and groups that show restraint tend to be more creative. However, if sexual freedom turns into anarchy, it can lead to a decline in creativity and societal issues. This cycle has been seen throughout history, like in ancient Greece and Rome.

So, to quote Gandhi again, "The future is for the nations that are chaste."[107]

CHAPTER XVII

The Risk Factors of Teenage Pregnancy

Teenage pregnancy has been a matter of public and policy attention in many developed countries for several decades. However, the nature and extent of this attention has varied across time and space, reflecting different social, cultural, and political contexts. In the final decades of the 20th century, successive British administrations began to perceive teenage pregnancy as a notable public health and societal challenge. This viewpoint was shared, to varying extents, by the governments of numerous developed nations. By the late 1990s, eight out of the 28 OECD countries were actively engaging in efforts to diminish instances of youthful conception, while an additional 12 nations considered teenage pregnancy to be a relatively minor concern (Unicef, 2001).[108] Within the United Kingdom, both preceding and following the ascent of the New Labour government in 1997, the matter of teenage pregnancy was deemed worthy of intervention. Notably, the British initiative aimed at addressing teenage pregnancy stands as an exemplar of one of the more sophisticated and enduring endeavors of its kind in the developed world.

Historically, marriage offered economic safeguards to mothers and their children, particularly during an era when the burden of unwed motherhood was primarily shouldered by local communities. Unmarried parenthood carried a significant stigma. In the late 1960s and early 1970s, a shift occurred in the United States, documented by Arney and Bergen (1984),[109] Furstenberg (1991)[110], and Wong (1997)[111], and slightly later in the United Kingdom (Selman, 1998/2001)[112] and other countries such as South Africa (Macleod, 2003)[113]. Public and policy concerns transitioned from the marital status of expectant mothers to their age, marking the emergence of the issue of teenage pregnancy.

The United States became seized with the issue of teenage pregnancy at an earlier juncture than the United Kingdom (Selman, 1998/2001).[114] By 1975, anxiety surrounding teenage pregnancy had become deeply ingrained in the United States. In 1976, the Alan Guttmacher Institute, a U.S.-based reproductive health organization, released its highly influential report, "11 million teenagers: What can be done about the epidemic of adolescent pregnancies in the U.S.?" The publication of this report not only popularized the use of the term 'epidemic' in connection with teenage pregnancy but also served as a catalyst for further policy initiatives.

In an introduction, Tony Blair said that the UK had the most teenage pregnancies in Europe. The authors mentioned in the first chapter that there are almost 90,000 pregnancies to teenagers in England every year, with about 7,700 to girls under 16, and three- fifths of them result in live births.[115]

A Unicef Innocenti Report Card (No. 3) in 2001 shared international data on teenage fertility. The report highlighted the highest rates among US teenagers (52 births per 1,000 girls) and the lowest in Korea (2.9) and Japan (4.6). While the US rates were high during the Unicef report, they were almost double in the early 1960s, with nearly 90 births per 1,000 teenage girls (Singh and Darroch, 2000).[116] The US, Canada, Australia, the UK, and New Zealand had higher rates of early pregnancy and childbearing than other developed nations (Chandola et al, 2001).[117]

Changes in teenage fertility are most noticeable in marriage trends over the past three or four decades. In 1971, three-quarters of teenage births happened within marriage, but by 2004, only 10% of teenagers giving birth were married. The decline mirrors trends in older age groups but has been steeper for teenagers. Nowadays, if a teenage mother is 17 or older, she's more likely to carry the baby to term and stay single or cohabit rather than marry. If she's under 16, she's slightly more likely to end the pregnancy through legal abortion than to give birth.

Before the 1967 Abortion Act, teenagers dealt with unplanned pregnancies through illegal abortion or adoption. From the late 1960s onwards, pregnant young women could legally terminate their pregnancies.

Reflecting the analysis in Teenage Pregnancy, popular media often portrayed early childbearing as a negative phenomenon, causing health issues, poverty, and educational failure. Young mothers' children were also thought to face similar challenges. Teenage pregnancy became strongly associated with social exclusion, a belief widely accepted at the time.

Over the next decade, as the Teenage Pregnancy Strategy was implemented and research on teenage pregnancy grew, the connection between youthful pregnancy and social exclusion became more prominent. Even with changing perspectives, teenage pregnancy is likely always to be seen as a problem in a world where fertility is deferred, education is prolonged, and economic independence is emphasized.

Teenage pregnancy is often linked to poor educational attainment or a lack of interest in education. Studies show that teenage mothers are more likely to have lower educational attainment scores at ages 7 and 16 than older mothers.

In popular belief, early parenthood is considered a cause of school dropout, although many young mothers leave education before pregnancy, sometimes due to bullying.

There's a common belief that young girls become pregnant to secure welfare benefits and council housing, especially scarce in some parts of the UK.

Analyzing Labour Force Survey data, there are differences in teenage fertility by ethnic group, with Black Caribbean, Bangladeshi, and Pakistani women having higher rates than White or Indian women.

Family structure's impact on teenage reproductive behavior is a consistent theme in research, closely aligned with socioeconomic status (lone-parent families are usually poorer than two-parent families).

In lone-parent families, the parent-child relationship may be more strained than in two-parent families due to less time and, consequently, a potential hindrance to positive family functioning. It's often observed that the daughter of a teenage mother is one and a half times more likely to become a young mother than the daughter of an older mother (SEU, 1999).[118]

Research from other countries confirms the relationship between teenage pregnancy and abuse in childhood. Psycho-social research links teenage sexual behavior, pregnancy, and parenthood to factors such as low self-esteem, emotional problems, and having an external locus of control. In BBC Online content analysis, nearly 60% of 162 news items focused on preventing teenage pregnancy.

Similarly, in Teenage Pregnancy, an analysis of 1997 data showed an estimated 87,000 children with teenage mothers in England and Wales. The number of teenage pregnancies rose again, reaching 42,200 in 2003, despite a costly government campaign to lower them (Daily Mail, 25 February 2005). According to a British MP, high teenage pregnancy levels create a 'vicious cycle of under-achievement, benefit dependency, ill health, lack of aspiration, poor parenting, and child poverty' (Daily Telegraph, 28 January 2008).

If the idea of teenage pregnancy as a calamity sounds too strong, consider research on the stigma attached to early pregnancy. Qualitative data from British teenagers demonstrated a belief that early pregnancy and motherhood could lead to 'social death' (Whitehead, 2001).[119]

The history of teenage pregnancy as an epidemic can be traced back to 1976 when the Alan Guttmacher Institute published the booklet '11 million teenagers: What can be done about the epidemic of adolescent pregnancies in the United States.' Seen in this way, teenage pregnancy becomes a dangerous entity that seems to have arisen from nowhere. Calamity spreads into personal, familial, geographical, and temporal spheres. It encompasses evils like welfare dependency, rampant sexuality, poor parenting, and residence in poor neighborhoods.

Teenage pregnancy can be intensified when placed next to other problems, creating a negative association with social or health phenomena. For example, juxtaposing teenage pregnancy with sexually transmitted infections (STI) can lead to viewing teenage pregnancy solely as a negative phenomenon.

The popularity of cohabitation increased, with 44% of births outside marriage in England and Wales by 2006. Of those, 64% were registered by parents living at the same address (ONS, 2007).[120]

In 1997, Prime Minister Tony Blair spoke about 100,000 teenage pregnancies every year, expressing concerns about the impact on families, education, crime, truancy, neglect of educational opportunities, and overall unhappiness. Later that year, Tessa Jowell, a prominent minister, announced an 'action plan' on teenage pregnancy, emphasizing the disastrous impact of unintended pregnancy on a woman, especially as a teenager.

Teenage Pregnancy was published in 1999, outlining government plans to address the issue. Tony Blair, drawing on the report's main themes, wrote a piece for the Daily Mail, expressing the belief that children should not be having children in a 'civilized society.' He emphasized that young people should not have sex before 16 and questioned the benefit of leaving a 16-year-old girl with a baby in her own flat.

Teenage pregnancy is often assumed to be a problem in academic and policy literature, much like crime, homelessness, and drug addiction. It's often considered a problem without extensive explanation.

Authors justifying concern with teenage pregnancy point to consequences in two main areas: alleged immaturity of teenagers and their economic dependency on others. These factors make teenage pregnancy both a socioeconomic and broadly defined health-related problem, leading inexorably to social exclusion.

Harsh Realities of Early Motherhood

Teenagers are considered not fully grown up yet, so having babies might not be good for their health or the health of their babies. It can make pregnancies harder, especially if the mom is dealing with anemia, smoking, or not eating well. Giving birth can also be riskier, with more chances of having a premature baby. Babies born to young moms might not be as healthy, with higher chances of being born too small or not surviving.

People think that because teenagers are emotionally less mature, being a mom is harder for them compared to older moms. Also, younger moms are more likely to feel depressed. This is what some studies suggest (Cunnington, 2001; Breheny and Stephens, 2007b).[121]

Talking about one serious issue, like having a baby too early, the research says: There seems to be a real link between teenage pregnancy and having a premature baby before turning 16. Most of the tiny babies born too early are the reason for more babies being born too small or not surviving. But the risks because of young age are not as big as those because of social, behavioral, and economic problems. Different countries show big differences. Sweden has a high ratio of teenage abortions – more than 1,800 for every 1,000 births to teenagers. Denmark is around 1,600, while in the UK, it's about 600.

In some Scandinavian countries, France, and parts of Eastern Europe, many teens choose abortion. In the UK, about 40% of teen pregnancies end in abortion, compared to 70% in Sweden. Abortion was crucial in keeping teenage pregnancies low in Sweden before 1975, and it still plays a big role. In Denmark, girls aged 15-19 are almost 40 times more likely to get an abortion than women 10 years older (Rasch et al, cited in Knudsen and Valle, 2006).[122]

A study in the 1980s looked at teenage pregnancy in 35 countries, showing how a society's attitude towards teenage sexuality played a big role (Jones et al, 1986).[123]

A review of programs in the US that promote sexual abstinence or abstinence plus other advice (since the 1980s) found: Some programs can change teens' behavior, but the effects don't last long. Both abstinence-only and abstinence-plus programs don't have a big impact on teens' sexual activity. But programs that teach about contraception do make a difference in what teens know and how they use contraception (Bennett and Assefi, 2005).[124]

When New Labour was in charge, the cost of teenage mothers was talked about, but not as the main reason to reduce teenage pregnancy. Instead, the focus was on the bad things that happen when people become parents too early. But one document from the Department of Communities and Local Government did say: Reducing teenage pregnancy makes economic sense. The NHS spends about £63 million a year because of teenage pregnancy. If a teenage mom doesn't find a job in the three years after having a baby, the government pays between £19,000 and £25,000 in benefits. Rough estimates say that every pound spent on the strategy saves about £4 for the public purse over five years. [125]

In both times when different political parties were in charge, they all agreed that teenage pregnancy was a problem. But the main reason given was usually about money. Children's Minister, Beverley Hughes, didn't agree with a study that said teenage pregnancy might be okay for some teens. She said it's not a good choice because there's lots of evidence that being a young parent is bad for both the mom and the baby (Daily Mail, 17 July 2006, p 25).

Teenage pregnancy is seen as such a bad thing that some teenage moms might get help even before their babies are born. Tony Blair said we can identify families where the kids might cause problems before they're born. He suggested that teenage moms and families with issues should get help to avoid problems. Blair mentioned that his government made big progress in helping with social problems but said there's still a group of people with lots of problems. He even talked about helping them before the babies are born (BBC News Online, 2006, emphasis added).[126]

In light of the myriad risks associated with teenage pregnancy, it is imperative to consider holistic approaches that can guide our youth towards a path of well-being and responsible decision- making. One such approach is the ancient practice of Brahmacharya, which, while often associated with celibacy, encompasses a broader philosophy of self-discipline and moderation in all aspects of life.

Brahmacharya encourages individuals to exercise restraint and cultivate a disciplined lifestyle, not just in terms of physical actions, but also through the regulation of thoughts and emotions. It is a call to prioritize long-term goals and personal growth over transient pleasures and immediate gratifications. For teenagers, this can translate into a focused commitment to their education, health, and the development of a strong moral character.

The practice of Brahmacharya is not about suppression or denial, but rather about channelling one's energy towards constructive and meaningful pursuits. It advocates for a balanced life where one is mindful of the consequences of their choices and actions. By embracing Brahmacharya, teenagers can develop the clarity and strength needed to navigate the complexities of modern life, while avoiding the pitfalls that can derail their futures.

In conclusion, as we seek to address the pandemic of teenage pregnancy, it is crucial to empower our youth with the wisdom of Brahmacharya. By doing so, we not only help them make informed choices that safeguard their well-being but also contribute to the creation of a more conscientious and resilient society.[4]

CHAPTER XVIII

The Challenges for Practicing Brahmacharya

I would like to express my anonymous view that practicing Brahmacharya in today's world is not easy because of various reasons. We live in a time of information overload, sensory stimulation, and social pressure. We are constantly bombarded by media, advertisements, and entertainment that promote sex, violence, and materialism. We are tempted by various forms of addiction, such as drugs, alcohol, gambling, and pornography. We are influenced by the opinions and expectations of others, such as our family, friends, peers, and society. We are also faced with the challenges of stress, anxiety, depression, and loneliness.

How can we overcome these obstacles and maintain Brahmacharya in our daily lives? How can we cultivate a pure and peaceful mind, a healthy and disciplined body, and a harmonious and compassionate heart? How can we achieve the ultimate goal of Brahmacharya, which is to realize our true nature and attain liberation?

In this chapter, we will explore the challenges and solutions for practicing Brahmacharya in today's world. We will discuss the various obstacles of Brahmacharya practice. We will also share some practical tips and techniques to help you practice Brahmacharya in your daily routine. We hope that this chapter will inspire you to follow the path of Brahmacharya and experience its transformative power.

The Power and Profit of Sex

I would reiterate, sex is one of the most fundamental aspects of human life, yet it is also one of the most complex and contested. How we understand, experience, and express our sexuality is influenced by a variety of factors, including biological, psychological, social, cultural, and historical ones. Among these factors, three industries stand out for their significant impact on our sexual culture: sexology, pornography, and pharmacology.

These industries, which we call the Sex Industrial Complex, shape our sexual knowledge, norms, desires, and practices in ways that are often hidden, controversial, and profitable. In this chapter, we will examine how the Sex Industrial Complex operates, what its effects are, and what challenges and opportunities it poses for sexual health and justice.

Pornographers and "sexologists," two groups who haven't been big fans of Judeo-Christian morals, values, and laws, have teamed up with "Big Pharma," a business with a lot of lobbyists and a huge budget for convincing people.[127] This trio wants pills for guys who have trouble in that area and a "Viagra" pill for girls. One sexologist said, "We've got what pharmaceutical companies want... they're looking for our help in making money... Pills for guys and a mood- boosting pill for girls might get covered by the new Medicare drug plan.[128] Our schedule is pretty busy now.[129]" Since about 58% of Medicare users at 65 and 71% at 85 are women,[130] if Medicare covers a pill to boost a guy's mood, it could make a ton of money. So, companies making lifestyle drugs want more women to be interested in feeling frisky. Because women have been holding back mainstreaming naughty stuff and the liberal sex ideas from sexology, all three groups now want to make girls and women more interested in being sexy. In the past, people might have called this a big corporate conspiracy.

As 94% of NIH scientists were found in a money-making connection with top officials, pocketing over $2.^{5} million from drug companies, even some lawmakers are involved.[131] This union between sex "researchers," naughty content makers, and drug companies is a big danger to national health and government. A first look at the Kinsey Institute "today" shows that around 95% of their money from the government, states, and companies goes into ways to make people more interested in naughty stuff.

They use naughty content in most of their experiments with students and others. So far, there are no reports of problems like addictions or obsessions from the experiments. But now, the law says lawmakers can get the names and addresses of everyone in the experiments, even if they promised to keep it secret. By calling themselves "health professionals," sexologists got academic credibility and the latest tech to test mood drugs and smells using brain scanners and other devices for studying sexy feelings.

There's clear evidence of a "money-making connection" between naughty content makers, drug researchers, and the Kinsey Institute (KI) led by Director,

Julia Heiman. Heiman also works for the "Sinclair Institute," an online naughty content seller that offers aids for naughty businesses, stuff like AIDS efficient "anal fun" devices called "sex toys." This public job fits with KI's history as a Playboy supporter, and their team is known for using, making, and being addicted to naughty content. About 95% of Heiman's money goes into making people more interested in naughty stuff, mostly by showing them naughty films. Even one small "cancer" experiment is about "Mood After a Short, Educational Chat." Another part-time study in 1999, "Boosting Recovery from Blood and Marrow Transplantation," wasn't listed on the National Cancer Institute or National Library of Medicine websites. It may or may not also check for naughty feelings.

Despite knowing that Kinsey's naughty child research was shady,[132] in 1998,KI boldly republished the Kinsey Reports (1948, 1953) as good and accurate science. In 2003, KI published Sexual Development in Childhood, using a bunch of questionable "experts" who either edit, support, or refer to naughty and even inappropriate manuals.[133] These KI child "experts" almost all say bad things about American morals and reject normal standards of being a kid and not knowing about naughty stuff. An ongoing attack on puberty (as the usual time for feeling sexy) supports KI's naughty child lies and the permissive sex codes from 1955 that started the current Naughty Content Complex. KI's experiments with sexy feelings match their Sexual Development in Childhood findings. Both support kids being interested in naughty stuff, which could mean a lower age for saying yes and more naughty content and mood-correcting drugs. What's normal for grown-ups quickly affects kids, with shots for child diseases and pregnancy already tested and two required (HepB, HPV) and more on the way. If health pros trained by sexologists control "mental health" screening and diagnoses (like in some Catholic schools), the future could be very worrying.

The Masturbation Industry: A Threat to Health, Relationships, and Society

What if I told you that there is a multi-billion dollar industry in America that is based on exploiting your natural sexual urges and turning them into a compulsive habit of self-gratification? What if I told you that this industry is supported by the government, the media, and the so-called experts who claim to know what is best for you? What if I told you that this industry is destroying the sacred meaning of sex, the foundation of the family, and the dignity of the human person?

In the way people think in the West, sex is seen as a way to achieve something. On the other hand, in a more secular viewpoint, sex itself is seen as the goal, and people in this view will use any method to reach that goal. Throughout the two thousand years of Western civilization, the main physical reason for sex has been considered procreation, and its social and spiritual purpose is seen as building a family. Therefore, it's meant for married couples, where it serves another purpose - bringing husband and wife closer, creating a strong bond that forms the foundation of a family.

Secularism, however, sees sex from a different angle. For them, the physical and social purpose of sex is, well, just sex. It's considered "natural." Interestingly, even though sex is viewed as entirely natural, those who follow this philosophy often work hard to manipulate nature. While advocating for artificial contraception, they essentially promote acts similar to mutual masturbation, turning intimate moments into a mere physical play. Whether a man spills his seed or uses a condom, there's no difference.

Now, you might hear experts, like doctors and psychologists, including past Surgeons General of the United States, saying that masturbation is good, wholesome, and healthy. But, in reality, they're not telling the truth.

In today's America, it's impossible to discuss sex without bringing up pornography, as it has become a significant part of our society. The sole purpose of pornography is to sexually arouse the viewer. It's a competitive market where the aim is masturbation. The U.S. government, which censors public Christian expressions, art, and education, protects and defends pornography as constitutionally protected speech. This has fueled the massive and growing Internet industry, driven by the demand for erotic content.

If you wonder about the most popular web pages today, it's not religious sites but rather those related to "adult entertainment," making billions in revenues. Cable networks, too, profit from "adult entertainment" TV, and even seemingly regular programming becomes more erotically competitive. Sports, fashion, and even music videos are becoming increasingly sensuous.

The economic boom of the Internet is heavily influenced by the demand for erotic content. People can engage in video "teleconferences" for sexual entertainment, contributing to the booming masturbation industry. Unfortunately, this trend also attracts individuals with harmful intentions, such as pedophiles and child pornographers.

Even seemingly "normal" industries and entertainment have jumped on the economic wave of masturbation. Mainstream TV becomes more erotically competitive, with talk shows discussing perversion and erotica. Fashions and popular music videos become increasingly sensuous. Prime-time sit-coms now promote and celebrate various illicit activities, pushing the boundaries in a media war against traditional morality.

It's hard to escape this trend. Even supposedly family-friendly channels like Fox News include advertisements for explicit content. The channels popular among kids, like MTV and VH1 feature videos with provocative content. It's not just adult entertainment; it's a market driven by extreme sexual arousal.

In conclusion, the content we are exposed to on TV, the internet, and even in everyday advertisements reflects a culture that seems to oppose traditional values. It's important for adults to be aware of what's being transmitted and take steps to protect children from exposure to adult content, which is often wrongly labeled as "entertainment." This goes against the values deeply rooted in Western Culture and the rich Judeo-Christian moral tradition.[134]

Sexualization of American Culture

In the book "The American Sex Revolution" by Pitirim Sorokin, the author delves into the profound transformation of American society regarding sexuality. This exploration unveils the intricate details of a significant shift in cultural attitudes and norms, shedding light on the evolution of American views on sex.

Over the past two centuries, and especially in recent decades, our culture has been strongly influenced by discussions about relationships. Sex is now a big part of American life and is visible in every aspect of our culture.

Literature: Our books often focus on sex, especially the more extreme forms of it. In the last century, many stories were about abnormal people— prostitutes, criminals, and those with mental health issues. There's a growing interest in the darker sides of society—broken families, unloved children, and the lives of criminals. Modern Western literature, aiming to capture readers' attention, often revolves around explicit portrayals of different types of love and engages in psychoanalysis of various psychological issues.

Music: The music has changed over time. In the 19th century, it was mainly religious or patriotic. But as we move into the 20th century, songs worldwide increasingly talk about romantic love, becoming more sensual and wild.

Stage, Movies, Television, and Radio: Entertainment, like movies, has also become more focused on sex. About 45% of movies in 1930 were about sex, and that trend has continued. Television brings explicit content into our homes, sometimes making us feel uncomfortable or dirty. The shows often feature passion and lust in their rawest forms.

Magazines: Magazines regularly show us pictures of attractive people and include erotic stories of all kinds. Even articles that claim to be educational often discuss topics related to sex, from Freudian theories to the intimate lives of historical figures.

Advertising: Advertisements now heavily rely on sex appeal to sell products. Whether it's a car, cosmetics, or food, you often see suggestive images. This trend is also present in radio and TV commercials, where both the ads and the programs themselves often have a sexual undertone.

Business: Businesses use sex appeal extensively in advertising, even though it contradicts moral standards. This dual approach may be undermining the moral and creative aspects of our society.

Science: Sex has even made its way into our sciences, influencing research in history, psychology, and sociology. While scientific research on sex is welcomed, there's a concern that excessive focus on sex in various disciplines is affecting our understanding of society, culture, and history.

Conclusion: The prevalence of sex in our culture is evident across various forms of expression. While some aspects of this influence can be positive, there's also a risk of it. Negatively impacting our society, from our understanding of relationships to our mental well- being.[135]

The Universal Theory of Madness

What is madness? Is it a disease, a disorder, or a deviation from the norm? Is it a curse, a burden, or a tragedy? Or is it something else entirely? Something that escapes the labels and categories that we impose on it? Something that reveals the hidden truths and possibilities of our existence?

In his Book "The Psychological Society", the author Martin L Gross has named it the theory of universal madness. We've started suspecting our friends, family, and even ourselves of having some mental issues. In New York City, a ten-year study called Mental Health in the Metropolis found that about 80 percent of adults showed signs of mental illness, and one in four had actual problems.

In 1977, the President's Commission on Mental Health agreed with these serious findings. It said our mental health is worse than we thought, and a quarter of all Americans are dealing with intense emotional stress. They warn that up to 32 million Americans might need professional psychiatric help.

A psychologist from the National Institute of Mental Health even sees universal madness as something very likely. "Almost no family in the nation is entirely free of mental disorders," he said in a recent federal study. He estimates that, in addition to the 500,000 schizophrenics in hospitals, there are 1.^{75} million psychotics not hospitalized, and up to 60 million Americans show weird mental behavior related to schizophrenia. He talks about the "psychological turbulence that is rampant in an American society that is confused, divided and concerned about its future."

Every year, millions get psychotherapy in many forms, from psychoanalysis to simple supportive therapy, either in groups or alone. Some look for Nirvana in the new wave of humanistic therapies, including many imaginative ideas from Gestalt Therapy to nude marathons. People are offered almost a hundred different psychotherapies, each claiming to be the best.

The outpatient psychiatric clinics are bustling with this new therapy trend. In 1955, they treated a total of 233,000 people. Since then, the number has risen a lot to 2.^{4} million patients annually. This doesn't include another 1.^{5} million patients treated each year in the 570 federally supported Community Mental Health Centers.

The main bases for psychotherapy are psychiatrists, most of whom see patients in their private offices, clinical psychologists, and psychiatric social workers (M.S.W. degree), the growing third rung of the helping professions. Based on a 1973 American Psychiatric Association study of private practice and a recent report from the American Psychological Association, we can estimate that one and a half million Americans get their psychic repair in the private offices of these practitioners.

In total, about six million Americans each year receive psychotherapy in clinics and hospitals and from private therapists. To get the complete number in therapy, though, we also have to consider the increasing number of lay therapists who offer a psychological inventory from est to primal workshops and encounter. At least a million more Americans get therapy from these sources, making it a total of seven million receiving psychological intervention annually.

This healing is not spread out evenly, as therapy professions have a geographical bias. Almost half the psychiatrists, for example, practice in New York, California, Illinois, Pennsylvania, or Massachusetts. Nearly one-third are in New York and California alone. But the profession is quickly expanding into the rest of the country. Even once psychologically isolated Nebraska now boasts over a hundred psychiatrists.[136]

Our world is filled with animals influenced by strong desires, including intense urges for intimacy and conflicting instincts related to pleasure and pain. In the United States, there is clear evidence of a focus on sex in various fields like psychology, psychiatry, sociology, education, and anthropology. This influence stems from the ideas of Freud, who believed in pan-sexual fantasies. Unfortunately, these theories have spread, affecting different areas of social sciences, leading to the acceptance of non-Freudian ideologies related to sex.

Despite the lack of scientific backing and the negative impact on essential human values like love, marriage, and parenthood, these theories persist. Many scientists and the public, including writers, artists, business people, government officials, teachers, preachers, and social workers, embrace these ideas. This success reflects a worrying trend of sexual obsession and mental deviation, affecting various aspects of our society. In terms of ethics and religion, hedonistic values promoting pleasure for the majority have gained widespread approval. Concepts like continence, chastity, and faithfulness are criticized as they supposedly deny pleasure. The focus is on justifying any enjoyable sexual relations, regardless of their nature. This shift in moral values has contributed to the loosening of societal norms, embracing premarital and extramarital relationships while dismissing traditional virtues like guilt and remorse.

The impact of this change extends beyond personal behavior. Beauty contests, parades, and entertainment industries now prioritize sex appeal for success. From fashion to cosmetics, the influence of sex is evident. Clothing designs, advertisements, and even daily conversations are saturated with sexual undertones. The rising tide of sex-mindedness has led to a progressive uncovering of the body, changing fashion norms significantly. Even our auditory, olfactory, and gustatory environments are not spared, as music, scents, and foods are designed to be erotically appealing. This pervasive sexualization of our culture has far-reaching consequences. Individuals, influenced by constant sexual stimuli, struggle to resist their overstimulated drives. Illicit relationships become more acceptable, and moral norms are disregarded. This shift in cultural values raises concerns about the well-being of individuals and the future of our nation. Addressing these issues requires a deep internalization of religious, moral, and legal norms to navigate the challenges posed by our sex-saturated environment.[137]

CHAPTER XIX

Why Brahmacharya Is Not Taught or Highlighted

First and foremost, it is evident that some fake sex experts have used this notion for their own profit and have instilled a fear of celibacy in the public mind, which is seen as a source of mental and nervous disorders and a serious threat to health. Based on this view, doctors and psychologists have blamed celibacy for the nervous problems of young people and have suggested young men to go to sex workers and expose themselves to sexual diseases as a preferable option than the supposed dangers of refraining from sex.

Secord, many people who aspire to follow Brahmacharya find themselves making excuses to avoid or compromise it. They may rationalize their indulgences, justify their weaknesses, or blame their circumstances. They may think that Brahmacharya is too difficult, too impractical, or too outdated for them. They may doubt its benefits, question its relevance, or fear its consequences.

I will examine the common excuses that people give to evade Brahmacharya, and we will expose the fallacies and delusions behind them. We will show how these excuses are the products of the ignorant and restless mind, which is enslaved by the senses and the ego. We will also reveal how these excuses prevent us from experiencing the true joy and freedom of Brahmacharya, which is the natural state of our being.

I will offer practical and effective ways to overcome these excuses, and to cultivate the attitude and the discipline that are essential for Brahmacharya. I will draw on the wisdom and the guidance of the ancient and modern masters of Brahmacharya, who have demonstrated its power and its possibility in their lives. I will also share the testimonies and the insights of the practitioners of Brahmacharya, who have discovered its beauty and its grace in their journeys.

The Causes of Brahmacharya Loss

Many people abandon the practice of Brahmacharya for various reasons. We will explore some of the scientific causes of Brahmacharya loss. Some of the main factors that lead to Brahmacharya loss are:

1. **Distractions:** You should identify the main sources of distractions in your life. Swāmi Vivekānanda advised to let your mind wander freely and observe it. After a while, it will settle down and you will realize that "I am watching my mind; my mind is separate from me". You will notice that your distractions have decreased, your mind has become calm and peaceful.

2. **Ignorance of potential:** Not knowing your potential is a major cause of semen loss. It leads to a lack of patience, courage, and ultimately, semen loss. You have amazing potential. You should recognize your potential and achieve success in your field.

3. **Excuses:** The person who does not want to work hard for his life makes excuses. He complains about his problems and situations, but the truth is that problems and situations improve your quality. It is not possible to do something extraordinary in a comfortable situation. Instead, people have done remarkable innovations in the most difficult and adverse situations of life. Stop making excuses and consider yourself lucky because you have been given challenges and human intellect. You can overcome all challenges with your effort and inner strength. This is the real joy of living a life.

4. **Irresponsible:** The person who avoids responsibilities is not able to have a strong mind power. His mind is always empty, which attracts evil and lustful thoughts. As a result, he loses semen. Responsibility is a better way to test our mind and intellect. It benefits individuals and those who want to follow the Brahmacharya Lifestyle.

5. **Misunderstandings of sex power:** One of the main reasons for excessive semen loss is a wrong understanding of sex power. Sex power is a very powerful emotion in a couple that creates new life. It changes into many forms. First, it changes into emotional attachment with children. Children have an emotional attachment to their parents. Then it becomes pure and changes into the emotion of siblings. Gradually it takes many forms of emotions. Nature cannot exist without emotional attachment. It is an illusion of "emotional attachments". A normal human is trapped in this web of emotional attachments.

Nature wraps up the creation inside the vast ocean of time, just like a spider makes a web that lives inside it and wraps it up. The wise man knows the importance of emotion and believes that beyond the illusion, there is full of bright knowledge free from all kinds of madness and distractions. The illusion will not affect the person if he wakes up in Brahma Muhūrta and practices yoga, meditation, and reads scriptures.

1. **Lack of spirituality:** We have already talked about the vital components of semen. Brahmacharya cannot be achieved only with scientific methods. We also need to use spirituality, which is a true science. Many eminent scientists and scholars have praised Indian spirituality. Indian scriptures and saints' books are very useful for anyone who sincerely wants to follow the path of Brahmacharya. You can only understand the essence of scriptures if you do spiritual practice every day.

2. **Food habits:** There is a saying - "Your food shapes your mind". Swāmi Vivekānanda has said, "Pure food leads to pure thoughts". Srīkrishna in Gīta advises proper eating and proper wandering. Vegetarianism is very helpful for Brahmacharya life. You should always eat Sāttvic food. Only Sāttvic food makes your mind clear and pure. Your mind becomes a wild animal and acts according to the false desire if it is not Sāttvic. But the mind becomes a tame animal that is very kind, obedient, and happy with Sāttvic food given by the master. You can be your own master by Sāttvic food. Then, practicing and progressing becomes very easy.

3. **Expecting results:** Some people expect positive results very quickly after practicing a few days, one or a few months of Brahmacharya. But they need to have patience and see the wonderful change that happens soon after they start following Brahmacharya. They should follow Brahmacharya Lifestyle for at least two years to see the positive change.

4. **Disappointment:** Disappointment is the main cause of overthinking and instability. When young men start overthinking about limited results, it causes anxiety. Negative thoughts increase and the man is tempted to ejaculate for instant pleasure. But that ends with bigger disappointment. And in this way, this cycle of semen loss speeds up.

Understanding why people struggle with Brahmcharya is key, but don't worry, it's not mission impossible. Embrace the Superhuman Brahmacharya Lifestyle, and not only will you tackle those challenges, but you'll also take charge of your body, senses, and thoughts to make the Superhuman Brahmacharya Lifestyle a breeze. Stay tuned for some awesome tips in our upcoming chapters.

CHAPTER XX

The Transformative Power of Brahmacharya Lifestyle

What makes a person successful, healthy, and happy? Is it money, fame, or power? Or is it something deeper and more subtle? In this chapter, we will explore the ancient concept of Brahmacharya, which literally means "living in harmony with the supreme reality".

Brahmacharya is not just about celibacy or sexual restraint, but about cultivating a disciplined and virtuous life that leads to mental, physical, and spiritual excellence. As the saying goes, "Like a strong base is needed to make a strong building, in the same way, good morals are the root of building a glorious personality".

Brahmacharya is based on the understanding that the human mind is influenced by various factors, both internal and external, that affect our thoughts, emotions, and actions. According to Napoleon Hill, the author of the classic book "Think and Grow Rich", there are ten mind stimulants that activate the human mind and shape our destiny.

These are:

- **The desire for sex expression:** This is the natural and powerful urge to express our sexual energy, which can be either creative or destructive, depending on how we use it.

- **Love:** This is the pure and unconditional feeling of affection and devotion towards someone or something, which can inspire us to achieve great things.

- **A burning desire for name, fame, and money:** This is the ambition and aspiration to attain recognition, respect, and wealth, which can motivate us to work hard and smart.

- **Music:** This is the art and science of combining sounds and rhythms, which can soothe, stimulate, or elevate our mood and mind.

- **Friendship:** This is the bond and relationship of mutual trust, support, and loyalty, which can enrich our life and make us feel connected and valued.

- **Mastermind group:** This is the alliance and collaboration of two or more people who share a common goal and vision, which can enhance our skills and knowledge and help us overcome challenges.

- **Mutual suffering:** This is the empathy and compassion we feel when we see others in pain or distress, which can awaken our humanity and kindness.

- **Auto-suggestion:** This is the self-talk and affirmation we use to influence our subconscious mind, which can shape our beliefs and attitudes and empower us to achieve our goals.

- **Fear:** This is the emotion and reaction we experience when we face a real or perceived threat, which can either paralyze us or push us to overcome it.

- **Narcotics and alcohol:** These are the substances and chemicals we consume to alter our state of consciousness, which can either relax us or harm us.

Among these ten mind stimulants, eight are natural and positive, while two are artificial and negative. Among these ten mind stimulants, the most potent and influential one is the desire for sex expression, which is the source of our sex energy. Sex energy is the creative force that drives all life and creation. It is also the force that can transform an ordinary person into a genius, if channelized in the right direction. A genius is someone who has mastered his or her mind and body, and has achieved extraordinary feats in any field of endeavor. A genius is someone who has a personal magnetism, a unique and positive identity that attracts and influences others.

How can we channelize our sex energy in the right direction and become a genius? How can we practice Brahmacharya in our daily life and reap its benefits? How can we differentiate between a normal person and a genius, and what are the qualities that identify a genius? We will answer these questions and more in the following sections of this chapter. Stay tuned and get ready to discover the secrets of Brahmacharya, the elixir of discipline and spirituality.

Here, we will explore how genius people access and use different sources of ideas and thoughts. There are three main sources:

- **The subconscious mind:** This is the hidden treasure that every person possesses, but only genius people can tap into it effectively. By channeling their sex energy to their subconscious mind, they activate it to a higher frequency and receive guidance throughout the day. They can have amazing and wonderful thoughts even in their dreams. Their decisions, work, and behavior become extraordinary.

- **The collective subconscious:** This is the pool of ideas and thoughts that other people have in their subconscious minds. Genius people can tune into this frequency and use other people's valuable ideas from afar. They use them wisely to achieve the highest success in their work.

- **The infinite intelligence:** This is the source of unlimited knowledge that transcends time and space. The ideas and thoughts of great people who have lived or are still living are floating in the ether. They are infinite and beyond imagination. Genius people can access these ideas through sex transmutation, which makes their ideas travel faster than light. They receive the idea, strengthen their thoughts, and put it into action. Genius people resort to this source when their own subconscious mind and the collective subconscious are not enough. Thoughts from the infinite intelligence are incomparable and 100% fruitful. They never fail as they are the most superior spiritual thoughts.

Now, let us understand the concept of personal magnetism, which is a quality of genius people.

- **Physical touch:** You may not feel anything special when you shake hands with a normal person, but you will definitely feel a positive impulse when you shake hands with a genius. This is a sign of personal magnetism. You will feel an instant enthusiasm that you may not have felt before.

- **Voice:** Genius people have a magical effect in their voice. Even if they are not musically inclined, their words have a musical melody and a captivating charm.

- **Movement:** Genius people are very active, regardless of their body structure. They walk with grace and serenity.

- **Sex transmutation:** Genius people are successful in sex transmutation, either consciously or unconsciously. That is why they have natural self-control or abstinence. They can connect their self-expression and emotions to their subconscious mind, and they do not try to impress others. Instead, their charisma spreads positivity among the people.

- **Appearance:** Genius people take great care to maintain their personality. They do not choose their clothing randomly, but according to their personality, body structure, and color.

The 50 Exceptional Benefits of Brahmacharya

What if we told you that there is a simple and powerful way to transform your life and achieve your highest potential? A way that can enhance your physical, mental, and spiritual well-being, and make you a genius in any field of your choice? A way that has been practiced and advocated by some of the greatest minds and souls in history, such as Swami Vivekananda, Swami Shivananda, Socrates, and Nikola Tesla? This way is called Brahmacharya, the yogic principle of self-control and discipline.

Brahmacharya is not just about abstaining from sex, but about channeling your sex energy, the most potent and creative force in nature, to higher and nobler pursuits. By practicing Brahmacharya, you can access and use different sources of ideas and thoughts, such as your subconscious mind, the collective subconscious, and the infinite intelligence. You can also develop personal magnetism, a quality that attracts and influences others. You can experience various benefits of Brahmacharya, such as increased energy, vitality, confidence, concentration, memory, intelligence, intuition, creativity, and happiness.

We will present the real success story of a young man who practiced Brahmacharya and achieved remarkable results in his personal and professional life. His name is *Prashil Parmar*, a 28- year-old engineer from Gujarat, who is passionate about social awareness and yoga & meditation. He will reveal the 50 exceptional benefits of continence that he experienced by following the Brahmacharya lifestyle.

Here are the 50 benefits of Brahmacharya that he experienced in his own words:

1. My mind is clearer and more focused. I have better concentration and memory. I feel peaceful and calm.

2. My heartbeat is steady and normal, even in stressful situations. I don't feel anxious or nervous anymore.

3. I don't feel depressed or sad anymore.

4. I don't have constipation or digestive problems anymore.

5. My joints are flexible and smooth when I run. My body is more agile and fit.

6. My eyes are bright and clear. I don't have dark circles under them anymore.

7. My body is full of energy and enthusiasm. I enjoy going out in the sun, running, and playing soccer.

8. I can use the power of my mind, body, and speech to achieve anything. I have unlimited potential and possibilities.

9. My concentration and comprehension skills improve. I can learn and understand things faster and better.

10. My willpower is strong and firm. I feel confident and capable of doing anything. I have control over my mind.

11. If I practice Brahmacharya for a few years with the right control over senses, my vital energy i.e. semen transforms into a subtle form and becomes more powerful.

12. My immunity is high and strong. I can fight off infections and diseases easily.

13. My physical, mental, and intellectual strength increases. I also gain more confidence and self-esteem.

14. I feel more joy and happiness in my life.

15. I respect myself and my values more. I have a positive self-image and identity.

16. I sleep less but relax more. I feel refreshed and rejuvenated every morning.

17. I have a high self-esteem and self-worth. I appreciate and value myself more.

18. I have a compassionate and empathetic attitude. I care and help others more.

19. I don't waste money on lingerie or uncomfortable undergarments. I save money and spend it wisely.

20. I have a habit of saving money. I plan and budget my finances well.

21. I have a habit of saving time. I manage and organize my time well.

22. I have a habit of saving physical and mental energy. I use and conserve my energy well.

23. Brahmacharya helps me to fight fatigue, general weakness, and nervous weakness. I feel more alert and energetic.

24. If I follow celibacy for a certain period, I feel a surge of energy within me. I feel more alive and vibrant.

25. Practicing Brahmacharya prevents premature greying of hair and many eyesight problems. I look younger and healthier.

26. Brahmacharya keeps my skin young, glowing, and wrinkle- free. I have a radiant and attractive appearance.

27. Controlling my senses saves my sperm which turns into "OJAS" and keeps me young. I have a youthful and vigorous spirit.

28. Brahmacharya has many health benefits, not just for spiritual persons but also for many Hollywood celebrities who follow the Brahmacharya lifestyle. I can be healthy and successful like them.

29. Brahmacharya helps me to control my anger and frustrations. I feel more calm and balanced.

30. I can focus well and eliminate all the clutter in my mind. I have a clear and sharp mind.

31.   It eliminates the risk of becoming a sex and porn addict. I don't have any unhealthy or harmful habits.

32.   The notion that something wrong might happen or I am less interested in sex by choosing this path does not hold. I have a healthy and natural attitude towards sex.

33.   I have a better understanding of the difference between love and sex. I don't confuse or mix them up.

34.   I understand that love is not limited to romantic relationships. I can love and be loved in many ways.

35.   Brahmacharya is devoid of any ill effects. It only brings positive and beneficial effects.

36.   Emotions of anger, ego, greed, and deceit slowly wither away. I have a pure and noble heart.

37.   My willpower increases so much that once I take up an idea, I am confident to make it happen. I have a strong and determined mind.

38.   I feel a rise of self-energy with the practice of Brahmacharya. I have a powerful and dynamic personality.

39.   I have better eyesight with continued practice and tolerance power. I can see and perceive things better.

40.   I can spend more time in front of my computer without my vision getting fuzzy and my eyes getting tired. I have a good and healthy vision.

41.   The floaters in front of the eyes also reduce or disappear completely. I have a clear and unobstructed vision.

42.   I have little or no fear. I don't worry about the future anymore. I have a confident and optimistic outlook.

43.   I can think and act calmly even in a dangerous situation without panicking and worsening the situation. I have a cool and composed demeanor.

44.   I start to feel real masculinity. I have a strong and assertive presence.

45.   I find it easier to remember things in a better way. I have a good and reliable memory.

46.   I can remember even old incidents and things that happened long times ago. I have a long and vivid memory.

47.   My mind becomes much sharper. I have a keen and intelligent mind.

48.   I don't have any worries about being caught while doing a certain act. I don't have any guilt or shame.

49.   I am wiser and not supporting crime or cunning activities. I have a moral and ethical conscience.

50.   I can control better other aspects of my life like food, exercise, etc. I have a balanced and harmonious lifestyle.

Many people have followed the path of Brahmacharya and achieved amazing outcomes. The only requirement is to begin and persist on this journey with resolve and diligence; then, luck will favor you. Continence is essential for the mind, body, and spirit.

Social and Spiritual Benefits of Brahmacharya

In the previous section, we discussed the benefits of Brahmacharya, but to experience some of the social & spiritual benefits, one needs to follow certain rules of the Brahmacharya lifestyle. One of the best things that one can learn from practicing Brahmacharya is self-discipline. Many young people lack discipline in their lives, which is essential for achieving their goals.

We understand that it is very difficult to resist sexual urges, and before we proceed, we want to emphasize that sex is more in the mind than in the body. If someone thinks about sex all day, he has problems with his mind or brain, not with his sexual organ. But if the same person realizes that sex is not an emotion or a true purpose of life and chooses the path of Brahmacharya for the next part of his life, he will learn real self-discipline. Once the individual learns how to control his mind and thoughts, nothing remains hard for him, as Brahmacharya is a supreme tool to unlock the door to his desired destiny.

It will help him with whatever he wants to do in life. Another benefit of continence is understanding what real love is. People feel depressed and anxious because they do not follow the Brahmacharya lifestyle. They do not know what true love is. When one grasps the real meaning of love, he becomes joyful, and it automatically eliminates almost all mental problems. When one knows what true love is, he becomes better at maintaining it. He knows how to live life overcoming all the emotional imbalances.

Last but not least, Spirituality - Direction toward God. Spirituality can enhance physical, mental, and emotional well-being. More religious or spiritual people can cope with stress better. This is not surprising, as spirituality in its various forms has been a source of comfort and relief from stress for thousands of years. Stress is the main cause of many chronic illnesses and mental health problems, such as anxiety and depression. Religion and spirituality have always been an integral part of human existence.

But because of non- continence, humans live an ungrateful and non- spiritual life. Spiritual wellness can benefit your body as well as your mind. Spirituality helps you by enabling you to find meaning in your life, which can lead you to greater happiness, feel more gratitude, experience more compassion, improve social connections and cope with stress better.

CHAPTER XXI

Eugenics Is A Divine Solution For Human Degeneration

In today's modern world, people are more concerned about the pedigree of their dogs, cats and horses but give no thought to how their children are conceived. According to a report from the Centers for Disease Control (CDC, USA), at least 50% of first marriages in the USA end in divorce (1.1% and rising in India), and 1.[2] million abortions are done annually (6-7 Lakh in India), 62% of women in reproductive age use contraceptive methods (50% in India) and 2/3rd of women in the USA have unintended pregnancies. In other words, more than half of all the pregnancies in USA are unintended! About 40 percent of births in the United States are to unmarried women.[138]

All this means a pathetic raise of unwanted progeny by disturbed couples producing disturbed children who grow up as disturbed adults and have disturbed families. Thus, overall the result is a disturbed society.

As per the *Vedas*, sexual union between the husband and the wife is not for sensual enjoyment but for the sole purpose of getting righteous progeny. *(dharmav iruddho bhutesu kamo 'smi bharatarṣabha).*[139]

In other words, each sexual act between husband and wife should be pre-planned for an auspicious day and time; prior preparations and a healthy regimen followed; and then with devotional consciousness progeny conceived.

Conceiving a child based on the principles of *Garbhadhana- samskara* determines whether the qualities of the soul attracted to take birth are demoniac or godly. Therefore, *Garbhadhana-samskara* is very important. As far as the sexual act is concerned, the Vedic scriptures conclude as follows:

evam vyavayaḥ prajaya na ratyaimaṁ visuddhaṁ na viduḥ svadharmaṁ

"Thus, the act of sexual union is prescribed for obtaining righteous progeny and not for sensual enjoyment. Foolish cannot understand this pure religion."[140]

Lack of Brahmacharya produces not only sick and weak children but also immoral criminals. Specifically, giving birth as a teenager is believed to be bad for the young mother because the statistics suggest that she is more likely to drop out of school, to have no or low qualifications, to be unemployed or low-paid, to live in poor housing conditions, to suffer from depression, and to live on welfare. Similarly, the child of a teenage mother is more likely to live in poverty, to grow up without a father, to become a victim of neglect or abuse, to do less well at school, to become involved in crime, to abuse drugs and alcohol, and eventually to become a teenage parent and begin the cycle all over again.[141]

In the big story of human life, making babies is like weaving an important thread for the future. The further discussion of this chapter is inspired from the book *The Coil Serpent* by C. J. Van Vliet and the American Sex Revolution Pitirim Sorokin is all about the connection between eugenics (making sure future generations are healthy and strong) and Brahmacharya (being mindful about our actions, especially when it comes to having babies). Let's explore why it's crucial to think carefully about having children to keep everyone safe and happy.

During the first stage of the American Sex Revolution, its leaders deliberately attempted to destroy marriage and the family. Free love was glorified by the official "glass of water' theory: if a person is thirsty, so went the Party line, it is immaterial what glass he uses when satisfying his thirst; it is equally unimportant how he satisfies his sex hunger. The legal distinction between marriage and casual sexual intercourse was abolished. The Communist law spoke only of "contracts" between males and females for the satisfaction of their desires either for an indefinite or a definite period,-a year, a month, a week, or even for a single night. One could marry and divorce as many times as desired. Husband or wife could obtain a divorce without the other being notified. It was not even necessary that "marriages" be registered. Bigamy and even polygamy were permissible under the new provisions. Abortion was facilitated in state institutions. Premarital relations were praised, and extramarital relations were considered normal.

Within a few years, hordes of wild, homeless children became a real menace to the Soviet Union itself. Millions of lives, especially of young girls, were wrecked; divorces skyrocketed, as also did abortions. The hatreds and conflicts among polygamous and polyandrous mater; rapidly mounted,-and so did psychoneuroses. Work in the nationalized factories slackened. The total results were so appalling that the government was forced to reverse its policy. The propaganda of "the glass of water" theory was declared to be counterrevolutionary, and its place was taken by official glorification of premarital chastity and of the sanctity of marriage.

Abortion was prohibited except, since 1945, in exceptional conditions involving the health of the mother or similar considerations. The liberty of divorce was radically curtailed; by the decree of July 14, 1944, it was made impossible for the vast majority of citizens.

By now the cycle has been completed, and a slight relaxation of this too severe repression of sex is making it moderately normal. Soviet Russia today has a more monogamic, stable, and Victorian family and marriage life than do most of the Western countries. Considering that the whole cycle occurred under a single regime, the experiment is highly informative. It clearly shows the destructive consequences of unlimited sex freedom, especially in regard to creative growth. In the period from 1918 to 1926, when that freedom was fostered, the Soviet government was preoccupied with destructive work, and the imprisoned Russian nation was unable to achieve much in the task of positive reorganization or creative cultural growth. After 1930, when the task of curbing sex freedom was essentially accomplished, the destructive activities of the government began to subside, and its constructive work gained momentum.

Increasingly fruitful were the efforts toward industrialization and economic growth, the building of the armed forces, the rapid development of schools, hospitals, and research institutes, the fostering of the physical and even the social sciences, and of the humanities. There followed a renaissance of the fine arts and literature, a notable decrease of the previous persecution of religion, and a restoration and glorification of the great national values of Russia, which had in the preceding period been vilified by the Communist regime.[142]

The Need for Morality: Making babies should be done with lots of care and thinking about what's right. Right now, sometimes people don't think enough about what's best for the babies that might come into the world. This chapter suggests that people need to be more careful and control when they have babies, putting the future of their kids first. The one imperative eugenic requirement is parental dedication to the child-to-be, even long before it is conceived.

Most parents are ready for any sacrifice, any renunciation for the well-being of their child, once it is born. But for its greatest possible well-being potential parents — and that means all youth — must be willing to keep their bodies in such a condition that a faultless seed and a perfect soil shall be available for the prenatal growth. Almost as a rule however the male contribution to the seed has been weakened, and very often infected with inheritable disease, by abuse of the reproductive organs. And where in the past at least the soil — the mother's body — used to offer the foetus a fair chance, this factor too is more and more exposed to vitiation. Mankind seems to deteriorate deliberately into animalistic parents of an ever more wretched posterity.

Any tampering with the sexual function before it is being used for the conception of a child endangers the purity of the seed and of the soil. Promiscuity is particularly fateful in this respect, because in the intimacy of the sexual act each of the partners leaves a permanent impression on the other. Traces of these impressions are carried to later partners, and eventually to descendants. Physical proof of this lies in "the recognized fact that for a white woman, when stamped with the sexual vibrations of other races, to bring forth a white child, even in conjunction with a male of the white race, is impossible."

Similarly, the prospective father brings with him the commingled, usually polluting influences of every woman with whom he has sexually conjoined. And these influences affect not only the physical constitution; they are much farther reaching in their effect, for "promiscuity in sex commerce adulterates the soul essences."' Therefore unbroken virginity of both prospective parents until they come together for intended propagation is an essential eugenic requirement.

Not less important for the progeny than sexual purity of the parents before intended reproductive action is the avoidance of ardent passion during coitus. For "carnal passions are transmitted...through conception in the fire of lust. The union of two bodies... need not be spoiled by vulgar sensuality, if a powerful affinity of souls imparts to it the ideal character of an appeal for their unborn child." A higher evolved ego can thus be attracted.[143]

Even a highly evolved soul like Paramahansa Yogananda could be attracted by self-restrained parents. Paramahansa Yogananda writes in his book "The autobiography of a Yogi, "Early in their married life, my parents became disciples of a great master, Lahiri Mahasaya of Banaras. This association strengthened Father's naturally ascetical temperament. Mother once made a remarkable admission to my eldest sister Roma: "Your father and I sleep together as man and wife only once a year, for the purpose of having children." [144]

Not only spiritually souls could be attracted by self-restrained parents, even creative geniuses, philosophers, scientists, thinkers, artists and writers could be born in self-restrained societies.

Let's explore how Greece before the second half of the sixth century B.C. had a strict code governing sexual life, which was confined to indissoluble marriage. All transgressors were punished, frequently by being outlawed from family and landed. At the end of that century, however, a moderate relaxation of legal and factual restraints became noticeable, and during the fifth and the first half of the fourth centuries B.C., this freedom continued to grow without degenerating into sexual anarchy. These same centuries are marked by an explosion of creativity in many fields.

This is the Greece of Socrates, Plato, and Aristotle in philosophy; of Polycletus and Polygnotus in painting; of Pheidias, Praxiteles and Scopas in architecture and sculpture; of Pindar, Aeschylus, Sophicles, Euripides, and Aristophanes in literature; Terpander, Simonides of Klos, Agathocles, Melanippides the Older, Phrynis, Bacchilides in music. The same period witnessed the greatest number of scientific discoveries and technological inventions made by the Greeks, (6 and 3 in the eighth and seventh centuries; 26, 39, 52 in the sixth, fifth, and fourth centuries; 42, 14, 12 in the third, second, and the first centuries B.C.). Finally, in the same period Greece reached the zenith of her political creativity and influence.[145]

Beginning with the second half of the fourth century B.C., sexual freedom increasingly tends toward anarchy; and during the third, second, and first centuries B.C., it spreads throughout the entire Hellenistic world. This same period witnesses a rapid decline of Greek creative genius in all cultural fields, accompanied by depopulation, demoralization, and the loss of political independence. A somewhat similar cycle occurred in Rome.[146]

The Role of Love and Thinking Ahead: Even when parents love each other, having babies doesn't always get the careful thought it deserves. But this chapter says that good parents should think a lot about what kind of kids they might have. It's not just about being in love; it's about making a loving choice for the children they might bring into the world.

Eugenics beyond Romance: Love is great, but for having healthy and happy kids, it's not the only thing that matters. This chapter tells us that even if there's no big love story, people can still have healthy babies. The key is that parents need to be dedicated to their future kids and take good care of themselves before having babies.

Important Rules for Having Healthy Babies:

Stay Pure Until You're Ready: Wait until you're ready to have babies before messing with the baby-making process. This helps keep everything pure and safe.

Be Pure Before Making Babies: Don't fool around with lots of different people before having kids. It can leave a lasting mark, not just on your body but on your soul too. Waiting and being pure are important.

No Hugs and Kisses during Pregnancy and Breastfeeding: Moms and dads need to avoid getting too close during pregnancy and when feeding the baby. It's better for everyone, and it helps babies grow up healthy.

Wait Until the Baby Stops Drinking Milk: Parents should wait until the baby is done drinking milk before getting close again. This is because the body produces something called prolactin that helps make milk but also tells us to wait before having more babies.

Avoiding Strong Feelings: Don't let strong feelings ruin the special time when babies are made. Keep the love pure, and don't let things get too intense during the baby-making process. The focus should be on a deep connection, not just physical desires.

In the journey of making sure our children are healthy and happy, combining Brahmacharya with eugenics is like following a wise path. It's about being smart and caring when it comes to having babies.

As the world changes, people in the future might look back and see that we learned to be more thoughtful and purposeful in bringing new lives into the world.[147]

CHAPTER XXII

Chakras - The Hidden Power of The Human Body

In this chapter, we delve into the fascinating realm of the conservation of vital fluid and its profound impact on the energy centers within the human body, known as chakras. As we embark on this exploration, it becomes evident that the act of conserving semen goes beyond a mere physical practice; it is a pathway to saving vital energy, the life force known as Prāna. The next part of this book will unravel the intricate connection between Prāna and the specific points on our body known as Chakras.

These Chakras, aligned along the spinal cord, serve as gateways for the flow of vital energy. There are seven such Chakras in the human body. As the saved energy ascends, it initiates the transfer of cosmic energy, referred to as Shakti, towards the head, culminating in what is known as Kundalini. In this chapter, we will delve deeply into the dynamics of Chakra and Prāna, understanding their significance in the Brahmacharya Lifestyle.

The term "Chakra," derived from Sanskrit, translates to "disc" or "wheel," symbolizing the spinning energy centers within. For optimal functioning, these chakras must be opened and balanced. Any imbalance or blockage can manifest as emotional or physical symptoms, indicating a lack of reserved vital energy required to ascend towards the head. The practices discussed in this chapter aim to unlock these chakras and embrace the Brahmacharya Lifestyle in its true essence.

Your spine is adorned with seven major chakras, stretching from the base to the top of your skull, although some experts suggest the presence of at least 114 distinct chakras in the body. The chapter further elaborates on the characteristics and significance of the seven main chakras:

What are the 7 Main Chakras?

1. **Root - Mulādhāra chakra (Red Colour):** The root chakra, or Mulādhāra, is located at the base of your spine. It provides you with a base or foundation for life, and it helps you feel grounded and able to withstand challenges. Your root chakra is responsible for your sense of security and stability.

2. **Sacral - Svadhisthāna chakra (Orange Colour):** The sacral Chakra, or Svadhisthāna, is just below your belly button. This Chakra is responsible for your sexual and creative energy. It is also linked to how you relate to your emotions as well as the emotions of others.

3. **Solar plexus - Manipura chakra (Yellow Colour):** The solar plexus chakra, or Manipura, is located in your stomach/navel area. It is responsible for confidence and self-esteem and helps you feel in control of your life.

4. **Heart - Anāhata chakra (Green Colour):** The heart chakra, or Anāhata, is located near your heart, in the centre of your chest. Unsurprisingly, the heart chakra is about our ability to love and show compassion.

5. **Throat - Vishuddh chakra (Blue Colour):** The throat chakra, or Vishuddha, is in your throat. This Chakra has to do with our ability to communicate verbally.

6. **Third eye - Ājnā chakra (Indigo Colour):** The third eye chakra, or Ājnā, is located between your eyes. You can thank this Chakra for a strong gut instinct. That's because the third eye is responsible for intuition. It's also linked to imagination.

7. **Crown - Sahasrāra chakra (Purple or White Colour):** The crown chakra, or Sahasrāra, is at the top of your head. Your Sahasrāra represents your spiritual connection to yourself, others, and the universe. It also plays a role in your life's purpose.

Additionally, the chapter explores the concept of Kundalinī, aiming to reconcile traditional theories with modern medical understandings of brain functioning. This journey involves a review of ancient concepts about

Kundalinī, shaped over millennia through practical experimentation, providing insights into this profound phenomenon.

What is Kundalinī?

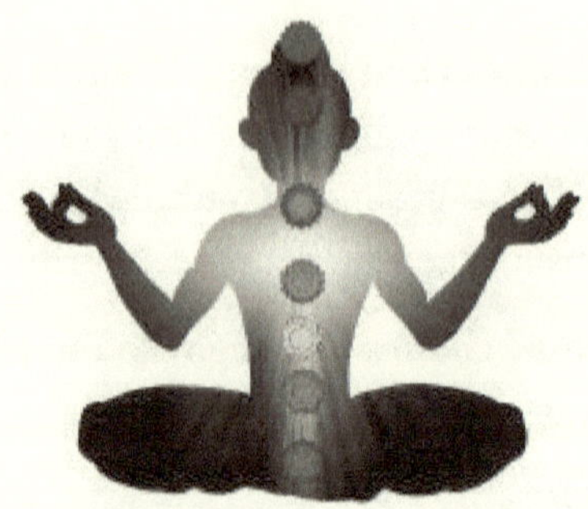

Let's figure out what it is by comparing what we know about how our brains work with the ancient ideas of Kundalinī. People thought about Kundalinī for a long time, like thousands of years. They tried things out to understand it, and that led to the ideas we have now.

The Science of Prāna and Kundalinī:

Ancient secret systems say our bodies are filled with smart, life- giving stuff. In India, they call it Prāna, in China, its chi, and Wilhelm Reich named it orgone. Different groups throughout history had their own names. This stuff connects our non-physical, spiritual side with our body, where we feel aware. Life needs energy, right? So, where does it come from? Think of it as creation having both still and moving parts, like Arthur Avalon explained. From a big-picture view, the still part is Universal consciousness, called Paramātmā or Shiva. The moving part is the first, creative energy making our physical world, known as Shakti.

Now, in humans, who are like small versions of the whole universe, Shiva and Shakti become our limited human awareness (jivātmā) and life energy (Prāna). Kundalinī is like our personal version of the big Cosmic Power (Shakti) that makes and keeps the universe running.

When our personal Shakti, acting as our own awareness (Jivātmā), joins the awareness of the top-notch Shiva, our world as we know it disappears, and we achieve Liberation (Mukti). Now, Prāna is pretty cool and creative. Let's take human reproduction as an example of its creativity. It's mind-blowing how a tiny fertilized egg turns into a full-grown human in just nine months – it's practically a miracle when you look closely. There are five types of Prāna in our bodies – Prāna, apāna, udāna, samāna, and vyāna. They seem like different roles the energy takes on to do things like breathing, digestion, circulation, and keeping our bodies healthy.

Where is this Prana Located?

The location of prana is hard to pinpoint, as it is very subtle and fine. No experiment has been able to measure it or fully understand its nature yet. Prana has two aspects. One is the individual prana, which is the life-force energy of each person. The other is the universal prana, which pervades the entire creation, from the energy fields of matter to the galaxies.

We all know that energy can neither be created nor destroyed (Law of Conservation of Energy). Prana is the name of this energy, which is abundant in the universe. In our body, prana is present in every cell, enabling it to function. The coarse form of this essence is extracted from the cells and tissues of the body and, through transformation, is converted into bioenergy, which powers the brain and the nervous system.

This energy is stored in the form of Shukra (Semen). Let us clarify this concept. Semen is accumulated in the Muladhara chakra (Bottom Chakra). This chakra plays a role in further processes. When someone preserves semen and follows Brahmacharya, this semen (Vital Energy, Kundalini) flows upward and gradually as it reaches the next chakra, it activates new chakras and reaches the Sahasrara chakra (Crown Chakra). There is a two-way flow of vital energy. A yogi knows when he wants this energy in different chakras. When the body feels sexual desire, this energy automatically travels downwards.

This is the cycle of Kundalini awakening. This is the most powerful process a person can experience in his lifetime. In Vedic culture, students practiced Brahmacharya from age 13 to 25 during their studies. That is why it was common to awaken their Kundalini then. But now, maintaining that long and pure Brahmacharya is very difficult.

What is pure Brahmacharya?

When we live in this polluted environment, it also matters that our vital energy that travels upward is pure. The quality and quantity of your vital energy affect the quality of your Kundalini awakening.

What if one awakens Kundalini by forcing the body or with impure energy?

When one tries to awaken Kundalini to its higher state just for energy and personal gain by forcing human nature or impure motives, first, it is very difficult to awaken Kundalini with impure energy or intention. But if someone does it, he will not have the joy of a good life. He will be unhappy and dissatisfied with this change in his body. His psychological balance will be disrupted, which may lead to insanity. Kundalini does not stay long in Sahasrara at first.

The duration depends on the intensity of the yogi's practice. There is then a natural tendency (Samskara) for Kundalini to return. The yogi will use all his effort to keep it above for a long time. He does this repeatedly so that it can be permanently fixed there. Kundalini is, therefore, a bipolar phenomenon, having the energy center at the base of the spine and the conscious center in the brain at the top of the spinal cord as the two poles.

What is Brahma-randhra ?

You are familiar with the concepts of Chakra and Kundalini awakenings. But do you know what lies beyond them? What will happen if we raise our Kundalini energy to its highest level? What will happen if we activate our Sahasrara (Crown Chakra)? This energy will reach Brahma-randhra. What is that? It is a center in the brain that is mentioned in some of the ancient East Indian esoteric texts as the Brahma-randhra, or the 'Chamber of Brahma'. According to *Gopi Krishna*, this center is the source of all the higher mental abilities that are related to the expansion of consciousness caused by the Kundalini awakening. Where is it located? It is the point where the canal from the spinal cord meets the brain's ventricles. This space and the ones around it are filled with the cerebrospinal fluid, which is said to be derived from the blood and similar to plasma.[148]

Brahma-randhra is a stable point that is difficult to maintain, but when the energy is high in Brahma-randhra, it is very hard to return to normal. There is a direct and immediate link between the basic mechanism near the genitals and Brahma-randhra in the brain. The stimulation of one also affects the other. The reason why meditation, which is a form of intense concentration, is so important in almost all spiritual practices is probably because of its activating effect on this center in the brain. The essence of yoga is concentration, and the last three steps, *Dharana*, *Dhyana* and *Samadhi*, are three levels of increasing intensity. In the final stage, Samadhi, the practitioner concentrates so deeply that they are unaware of any external stimuli. The relationship between concentration and the brain is further supported by the fact that many people who have trouble during intense Kundalini activity report a direct connection between the degrees of mental distress they feel and the amount of concentration they do.

If it is true that the energy going to the brain during Kundalini activity is mostly coming from the sexual organs, then any use of this energy for physical purposes will also reduce the available supply for powering the conscious center. Interestingly, many cases of Kundalini awakening have reported a partial or complete loss of sexual desire.

The aim of telling you all this science of Brahma-randhra is not to make you feel sad or regretful that you have spent much time without knowing this science. The main goal is to awaken you to the amazing benefits of Brahmacharya. When one starts meditating as part of his lifestyle, he starts living the life of a superhuman. You connect with the universal cosmic energy when your maximum energy is in Brahma-randhra. Do not make this process artificial. The best way to find purpose in life is this. Make this process natural so that you have no mental issues after this happens.[149]

Mirror Neuron Principle for Brahmacharya

We have already learnt more than enough about Brahmacharya, but why do some people abandon this path and resume their sexual life? The main reason is that they feel some inner discomfort or emptiness, a loneliness in their soul, and they think that Brahmacharya is not suitable for them, so they give up. Another important reason is related to the science of habits.

Before we learn how habits are formed, let us understand how the body and brain work. The brain is full of nerve cells, which make it very fast. Many scientists have shown that the brain uses electrical signals to function at high speed. When we want to do any task, we first send a signal to the brain nerves, which then transmit it to the body and also within the brain.

According to Donald Hebb, the brain creates a pattern when it repeats the same task. For each task, there is a specific pattern of brain neuron activity that completes the task. When we start or stop any habit, the pattern of the brain changes and adapts to the new situation. For example, if there are two options, one of drinking wine and one of not drinking, and we form a habit of drinking wine, then that option will become more prominent and strong, and the other option of not drinking will gradually fade away and disappear.

Hebb's law states that "Neurons that fire together wire together."

Mirror Neuron Principle: This principle states that physical restraint alone is not enough for Brahmacharya, because thoughts can also trigger neuronal activity. When scientists observed the brain signals of monkeys eating bananas, they found that the same signals were present in monkeys who were just watching another monkey eat a banana. This means that when we merely see or think about sexual thoughts, we are still violating Brahmacharya.

People who aspire to practice Brahmacharya

1. **The Ignorant:** They have no knowledge; they do not want to improve themselves and prevent others from doing so. They are lazy, ignorant, and think they are already right about life.

2. **The hedonist:** They follow two contradictory principles of life. They want to enjoy the benefits of Brahmacharya and also indulge in sexual feelings. They include No-Fappers and those who seek to cure PE (Premature Ejaculation) or ED (Erectile Dysfunction).

3. **The "Theory masters" but "Practical Failures":** They have knowledge but not wisdom. They cannot live the lifestyle they desire. They do not perform all the actions that are necessary for Brahmacharya. The reason for this lies in Hebb's law. They cannot change their habits of masturbation and sexual desires. Their brain neurons are fixed in such a way that they get disturbed and start altering their patterns. But they need to change their brain circuit by practicing new patterns. They cannot think about great sex, wet dreams, and desires while they want to live a Brahmacharya life. They can only purify

the dirty water in a glass by pouring more clean water into it, which will eventually clear the water; similarly, changing old habits takes time and requires constant input of positive thoughts.

4. **The Superhuman:** They know and have the wisdom to follow the path. They are practicing true Brahmacharya in life. They also help others to become like them. All other physical problems are healed when you start following this lifestyle. You do not have to worry about these problems. Just practice daily to strengthen the new pattern of brain activity. In the next chapter, you will learn all the practices that are essential for rewiring the brain firmly to the pure path of Brahmacharya.

CHAPTER XXIII

How to follow the Superhuman Brahmacharya Lifestyle

You might be interested in the rules of Brahmacharya after learning about its benefits. To practice Brahmacharya, you need to follow some guidelines that will help you achieve its advantages. If you follow these guidelines faithfully and sincerely, you will have no doubts or regrets. Let me tell you a story before I reveal these guidelines.

There was a man who was sailing in a boat. His boat hit many large rocks and stones on the way. These stones created 25 holes in his boat. He managed to seal 24 holes, but he left one hole open. His boat eventually sank into the river. Why? Because one hole is enough to sink the boat.

Likewise, to succeed in Brahmacharya or semen retention, you have to follow these 25 rules in your life, and you will never fail in your Brahmacharya. This is not my opinion, but the experience of great scholars who practiced Brahmacharya.

1. **Firm Resolve:** Scriptures and wise counsel affirm that confidence yields results. Therefore, before sleep and upon awakening, cultivate thoughts of courage, divine empowerment, valor, self-assurance, and boundless capability. Recall the Bhagwat Gītā's verse: " Sanshayātmā Vinashyati" - Those who doubt are doomed, thus maintain a positive mindset.

2. **Purified Perception:** Recognize that distorted vision is the root of many troubles. Reframe your outlook to view every woman as a revered figure, akin to a mother or sister. Should inadvertent sights occur, swiftly redirect your thoughts to maternal reverence. Practice averting your gaze when conversing with women to safeguard against impure fantasies, thereby preserving Brahmacharya.

3. **Simplicity in Living, Nobility in Thought:** Eschew excessive pursuit of fashion, as it detracts from true well-being. The abundance of food tempts false hunger, leading to indulgence even when unnecessary.

Shun environments and associations steeped in lust, opting instead for a modest lifestyle to shield against its destructive influence.

4. **Shun Negative Influence:** Beware the perils of bad company, which corrodes character and behavior. Just as a snake bite is fatal, repeated exposure to detrimental influences gradually erodes moral fiber. Choose association wisely, for it shapes one's persona and environment, leading either to spiritual elevation or moral decay.

5. **Regular Scriptural Study:** In the absence of virtuous companionship, turn to scriptures for guidance and inspiration. Engage daily with the wisdom of great souls, finding therein solutions to life's myriad challenges.

6. **Physical Purity, Mental Clarity:** A clean body is a prerequisite for Brahmacharya. Therefore, prioritize thorough cleansing through proper bathing rituals.

7. **Dietary Discipline:** The link between Brahmacharya and diet is profound. Overeating invites the wrath of the God of Sex, hindering the pursuit of Brahmacharya. Embrace a simple, Sāttvic diet, consuming in moderation to nourish both body and mind.

8. **Renounce Toxic Habits:** Abandon all forms of intoxication and addiction, as they dilute resolve and impede progress towards Brahmacharya. Maintain vigilance over health by eschewing alcohol, smoking, and similar vices.

9. **Combat Constipation:** Recognize that excessive seminal loss often stems from unresolved constipation. Prioritize regular bowel movements to uphold bodily health and vitality.

10. **Genital Hygiene:** Adhere to meticulous cleanliness practices, particularly after urination and bathing, to safeguard reproductive health.

11. **Embrace Physical Activity:** Regular exercise fortifies the body, rendering it less susceptible to illness. If unable to engage in structured exercise, prioritize brisk walking to invigorate both body and mind.

12. **Early to Bed, Early to Rise:** Commence each day with diligence, for the morning heralds boundless opportunities. Embrace the tranquillity of early hours, establishing a routine of spiritual and physical disciplines.

13. **Harness the Power of Prānāyāma:** Cultivate inner strength and vitality through disciplined breath work, which fosters physical well-being and mental equanimity.

14. **Embrace Fasting:** Regular fasting purges impurities from the body, promoting physical health and spiritual elevation in accordance with ancient wisdom. Fasting once in a fifteen days is strongly recommended.

15. **The Potency of Vows:** Uphold noble vows with unwavering resolve, for they serve as bulwarks against temptation and reinforce the commitment to Brahmacharya.

16. **Maintain a Diary:** Document daily reflections to cultivate self-awareness and accountability, fostering personal growth and adherence to Brahmacharya.

17. **Conquer Laziness:** Busy yourself with virtuous pursuits to stave off lethargy and temptation, thereby upholding the principles of Brahmacharya.

18. **Uphold Righteousness:** Adhere steadfastly to one's prescribed duties, for righteousness forms the bedrock of moral integrity and spiritual advancement.

19. **Cultivate Consistency:** Align daily routines with the natural order to foster physical, mental, and spiritual well-being, thereby fortifying the resolve to uphold Brahmacharya.

20. **Utilize Protective Garments:** Employ the traditional practice of wearing a *langot* to safeguard against seminal loss and maintain mental tranquillity.

21. **Harness the Power of Khadāu:** Embrace the benefits of wearing Khadāu, which exerts pressure on vital nerves, preserving Brahmacharya and spiritual vitality.

22. **Moderate Luxury:** Exercise restraint in indulgence, for excessive luxury undermines spiritual fortitude and erodes the pursuit of Brahmacharya.

23. **Fear of Public Disgrace:** Let the prospect of societal censure serve as a deterrent against actions detrimental to Brahmacharya, thereby preserving honour and dignity.

24. **Cultivate Devotion:** Nurture spiritual devotion as a means of purifying the mind and fortifying resolve in the pursuit of Brahmacharya.

25. **Comprehensive Adherence:** Integrate these principles into daily life with steadfast dedication, for their collective practice promises transformative growth and fulfilment of Brahmacharya.

Above are the guidelines to make living the Superhuman Brahmacharya lifestyle simpler. Let's explore different ways to follow these 25 rules of Brahmacharya effortlessly and stress-free.

CHAPTER XXIV

Yogasana And Pranayama for Brahmacharya

Yogasana for Brahmacharya constitutes a vital component of the superhuman lifestyle. Merely practicing Brahmacharya at the mental and spiritual levels is insufficient; one must also embody Physical Brahmacharya through Yogasana. Referenced is a Vaisheshika Sutra penned by the ancient sage Āchārya Kanād around 600 BCE, which echoes Newton's First Law, stating, "Vegah Nimittavesheshāt Karmno Jāyate." This law, analogous to Newton's principle, asserts that an object remains at rest or in motion unless acted upon by an external force. Similarly, within the context of Brahmacharya Lifestyle, adhering to this law implies that adopting Brahmacharya alone enables one to surmount physical, mental, and behavioral challenges. The prescribed Yogasana for Brahmacharya outlined here constitutes a fundamental aspect of the transformative Superhuman Brahmacharya Lifestyle. Neglecting this crucial element often leads individuals to falter in their Brahmacharya practice prematurely.

Remember: Prior to engaging in Āsanas, it's essential to recognize that just as you cannot see your reflection clearly in a dirty mirror, your biological and psychological systems may be tainted by negative influences. Thus, cleansing these systems is paramount.

Through the practice of Āsanas and following the guidelines outlined in the book, you can detoxify your being. Consistent practice, especially during the "Brahmamuhūrta," will imprint positive impressions in your subconscious, gradually integrating them into your daily life. This positive outlook towards Brahmacharya will attract favorable circumstances. Remember, you're not just cultivating a habit; you're shaping your character, a process that requires time but yields invaluable rewards. The following Yogāsanas will aid in internal cleansing, particularly strengthening the muscles surrounding the pelvic area, thereby enhancing sexual vitality and improving overall nervous system function. Start by warming up your body for 20 minutes upon waking or engaging in light exercise. Performing these Āsanas after your morning bath will yield remarkable results, facilitating both physical and mental well- being, and paving the way for meditation. Let's embark on our Yogāsana practice now.

Pādapashchimottāsana:

Method: Start in Staff Pose (Stretching your legs out of the body), sitting on the edge of a folded blanket. Push your heels away from your body; press your palms or fingertips into the floor next to your hips.

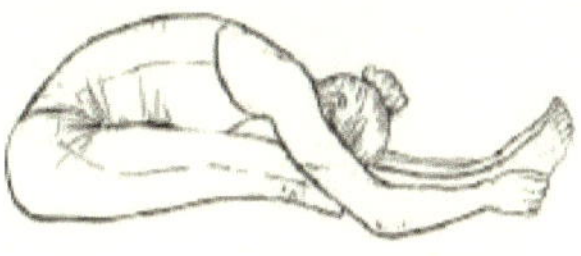

Pādapashchimottāsana

Inhale. Keep your front torso long, exhale, and bend forward from your hips. Extend the spine to fold over your legs without curving your back. Move your hands out along the outside of each leg as far as they can go. If you can reach them, grab the sides of your feet with your hands. With each inhalation, raise and extend your front torso slightly; relax more into the forward bend with each exhalation. If you are holding your feet, bend your elbows to the sides and lift them off the floor. Stay in the pose for 1–3 minutes. To come up, let go of your feet. Inhale and raise your torso by pulling your tailbone down and into the pelvis.

Benefits: This Asana purifies the nerves, which helps enhance one's working capacity and cures many diseases. Helps to cure various physical disorders like indigestion, constipation, common cold, acute coryza, productive cough, backache, hiccups, leukoderma, urinary diseases, wet dreams, seminal disorders, appendicitis, sciatica, urethritis, jaundice, insomnia, asthma, hyperacidity, nervous debility, uterine disorders, menstrual irregularity, impotence (sterility), blood-related disorders, stunted growth, and many other diseases are cured by this Asana.

Brahmacharyāsana:

Method: Sit on your knees on the mat. Extend the legs on both sides with both hands on the knees. Place your bottom on the ground between both legs. Keep your eyes in front and sit calmly. Practice this Āsana for 5 to 10 minutes before sleeping, repeating the Mantra *"Om Aryamāye Namah"* with Faith while doing this Āsana gives special benefits.

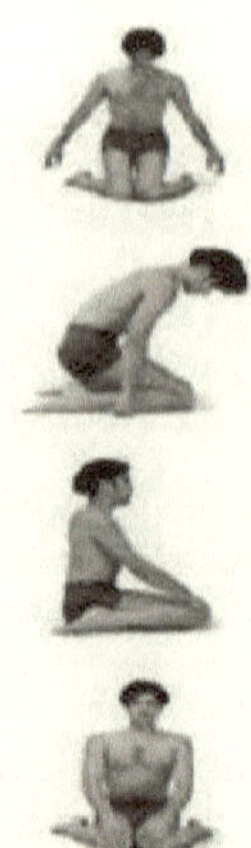

Brahmacharyāsana

Benefits: It helps in maintaining the defected organ area. It helps in controlling sexual impulses, making them flow upwards. It reduces the heat in nerves. Reduces the problems like wet dreams. It strengthens our Brahmacharya. It keeps our stomach clean.

Mayurāsana:

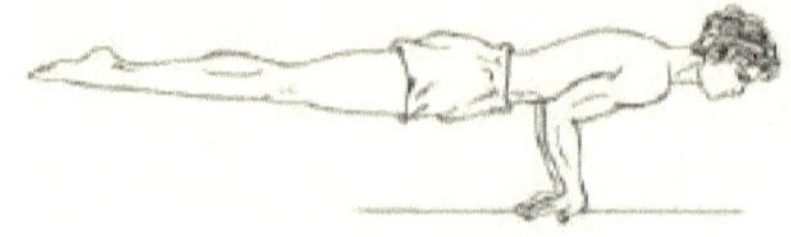

Mayurāsana

Method: Kneel on a carpet. Place your hands on the ground, pointing toward your feet. Bend both elbows, resting them near your belly button. Now lean your body forward and stretch your legs backward. Exhale, lift both legs from the ground and lower your head, so your body is parallel to the ground. The elbows support the weight of your whole body. While doing this Āsana, focus on Manipura Chakra. Stay in the position as long as you can. Then slowly return to the original position.

Benefits: Mayurāsana is very good for Brahmacharya. It strengthens your palms and arms. It helps diabetic patients a lot. It improves blood circulation in the body; thus all body organs become strong and effective.

Caution: People with high blood pressure and hernia should avoid this Asana.

Supta-Vajrāsana :

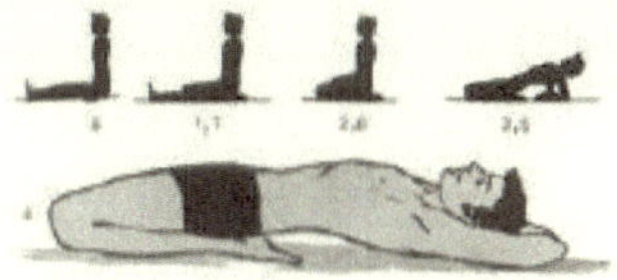

Supta-Vajrāsana

Method: Sit in Vajrasana with both thighs together and lie down on your back. Keep both your thighs together. Now, exhale, put your left hand under the right shoulder and your right hand under the left shoulder. Keep your head above the cross formed by your hands. Do Tribandh after exhaling. Focus on Vishuddh Chakra.

Benefits: It relaxes your Spinal cord. It makes all inner glands strong. It boosts your appetite and clears painful, hard stools. It also helps with Wet Dreams, Semen diseases, stones, deafness, eye weakness, tonsils, etc.

Sarvāngāsana:

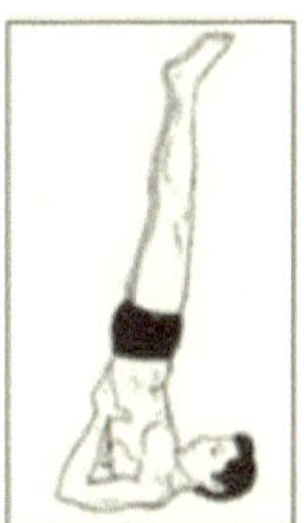

Sarvāngāsana

Sarvāngāsana is a Sanskrit word, with Sarv, which means the whole anga, which means all your body parts, and 'āsana,' an exercise. When you do this Āsana, your body is involved; you lie on your back and then raise your legs to a 90-degree angle. Then you lift your hips off the ground with your hands to support them and balance your whole body on your shoulders.

Method: Exhale, straighten your legs and align them with your body. Keep your knees straight and your body above the hip joint on the ground steady. Exhale, lift your arms, hold your waist and lift your body as high as you can. Put all your body weight on your arms and rest them on your elbows, keeping your legs vertical. Once you are stable in this position, slowly move your hands toward your waist with your fingers pointing to the back of your hip bones and your thumbs lightly pressing on either side of your navel. Tuck your chin into the jugular notch, then put all your weight on your shoulders, neck, and side of your head (final posture). You can finish this process within 4 seconds of inhaling. Stay in this pose as long as you are comfortable, but not more than two minutes, then breathe in a rhythmic, slow, and natural way. Please return to the starting position. Gently bend your knees, then lower them to the mat. Support them with your hands for 4 seconds, inhaling. Release your hands from your back and resume the initial position. Take several deep breaths, and rest for a few minutes.

Benefits: Improved vasomotor function (related to the widening or narrowing of blood vessels) due to the increased blood exchange in the upper part of our body, especially the neck, chest, and head. Temporary relocation of pelvic and abdominal organs. Remarkable effects of gravity pressure on the various body organs above the waist, including the vital endocrine glands. Relief for constipation, headache, indigestion, nerve pain, and neurasthenia. Neurasthenia is a functional disorder in the eyes, ears, throat, nose, and general sexual health. Increased blood flow to the brain. Balanced respiratory, circulatory, and digestive systems, as well as reproductive and nervous systems, and enhanced immune system. Increased flexibility of the cervical spine, which positively affects the nerves. Reduced lower abdominal sagging by toning the muscles. This can also help to avoid hernias. Reduced haemorrhoids by relieving the gravitational pressure of the anal muscles. Alert mind, which boosts self-confidence.

Surya Namaskāra:

Surya Namaskāra, or Sun salutation, is a series of 12 powerful yoga poses. It is not only a great cardiovascular workout, but also a way to impact the body and mind profoundly. The best time to practice Surya Namaskāra's steps is early in the morning on an empty stomach. Each round of Sun salutation consists of two sets, each with 12 yoga poses. You may find different versions of how to do the Sun salutation. However, it is advisable to stick to one particular version and practice it regularly for the best results. Sun rays have anti-bacterial and sterilising effects. Surya Namaskāra also gives you a chance to express gratitude to the sun for supporting life on this planet. Surya Namaskāra has amazing spiritual benefits. It is good for skin diseases because when you thank the sun, you receive positive energy for a better mental and physical state.

Benefits of Surya Namaskāra: It helps in losing weight and helps to keep you healthy and free from diseases. Balances the body and mind Improves blood circulation and digestion system. Strengthens the heart and lowers stress level. Stimulates abdominal muscles, respiratory system, lymphatic system, spinal nerves, and other internal organs Tones the spine, neck, shoulder, arms, hands, wrist, back, and leg muscles, thereby improving overall flexibility Psychologically, it regulates the connection of the body, breath, and mind It makes one calm and boosts energy levels with sharpened awareness. It helps treat insomnia naturally. Helps in skincare and hair care.

12 Steps of Surya Namaskar:

1. Pranāmāsana (Prayer pose):

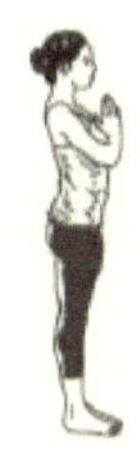

Stand at the edge of your mat, keep your feet together and balance your weight equally on both feet. Expand your chest and relax your shoulders. As you breathe in, bring your palms together in front of the chest in a prayer position.

2. Hasta Utthānāsana (Raisedarmspose):

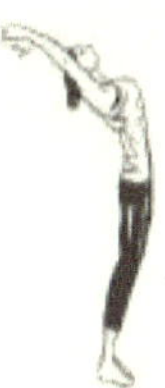

Breathing out, raise the arms up and back, keeping the biceps close to the ears. In this pose, the aim is to stretch the whole body up from the heels to the tips of the fingers.

3. Pādahastasana (Standing forward bend):

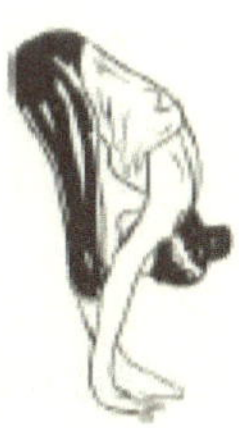

Breathing in, bend forward from the waist, and keep the spine straight. Bring your hands to the floor beside your feet as you inhale fully. Tip to deepen this yoga stretch: If needed, you may bend the knees to bring the palms down to the floor. Now try to straighten the knees gently. It's a good idea to keep the hands in this position and wait to move them until we finish the sequence.

4. Ashwa Sanchalanasana (Equestrian pose):

Breathing out, move your right leg back, as far back as you can. Bring the right knee to the floor and look up.(*Tip to deepen this yoga stretch: Make sure that the left foot is exactly in between the palms).*

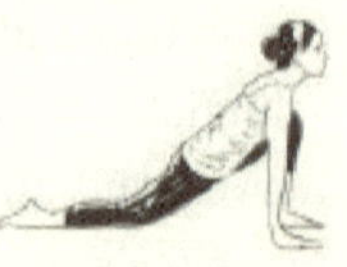

5. Parvatāsana (Downward facing dog pose):

Breathing in, lift the hips the tailbone to bring the body and into an inverted 'V' pose.(Tip to deepen this yoga stretch: Keep the heels on the ground and gently lift the tailbone, going deeper into the stretch)

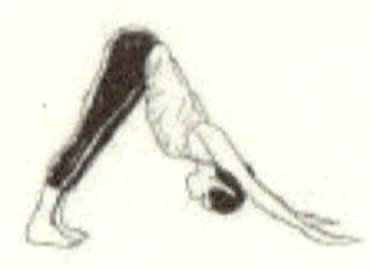

6. Ashtanga Namaskara (Salute with eight parts or points):

Breathing out, gently bring your knees down to the floor and inhale. Take the hips back slightly, slide forward, and rest your chest and chin on the floor.

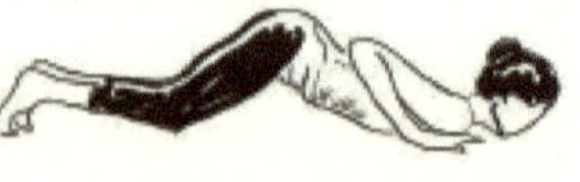

Lift your posterior a little bit. The two hands, feet, knees, chest and chin (eight body parts) should touch the floor.

7. Bhujangasana (Cobra pose):

Slide forward and lift the chest into the Cobra pose. Inhale deeply and keep your elbows bent in this pose with the shoulders away from the ears. Look up at the ceiling. (Tip to deepen this yoga stretch: As you inhale, try to push the chest forward gently; as you exhale, try to push the navel down gently. Tuck the toes under. Make sure you're stretching as much as you can and not forcing your body).

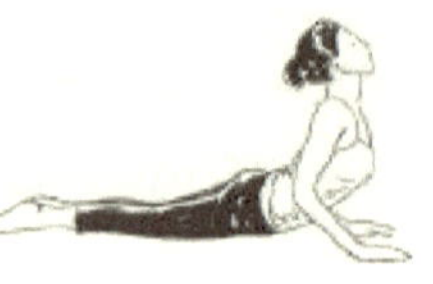

8. Parvatāsana (Downward facing dog pose):

Exhale, raise the hips and the tailbone to bring the body into an inverted 'V' pose. Tip to deepen this yoga stretch: Keep the heels on the ground and gently raise the tailbone, going deeper into the stretch

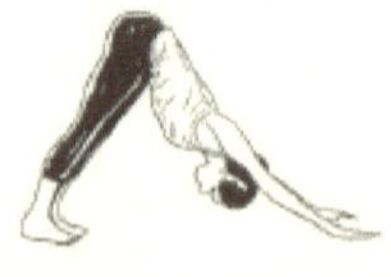

9. AshwaSanchālānāsana (Equestrian pose):

Inhale, move the right foot forward between the two hands. The left knee touches the floor. Lower the hips and look up. Tip to deepen this yoga stretch: Put the right foot exactly between the two hands and the right calf vertical to the floor. In this position, try to lower the hipstowards the floor gently, to deepen the stretch.

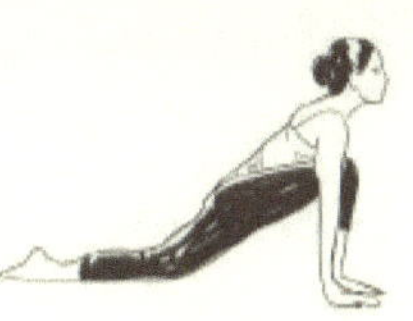

10. Padahastāsana (Standing forward bend):

Exhale, bring the left foot forward. Keep the palms on the floor. You can bend the knees if needed. Tip to deepen this yoga stretch: Slowly straighten the knees, and if possible, try and touch your nose to the knees. Keep breathing.

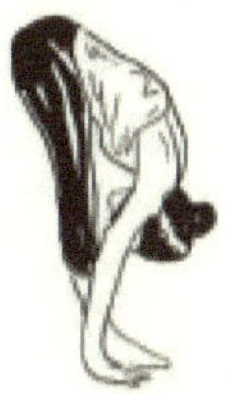

11. Hasta Uttānāsana (Raised arms pose):

Inhale, roll the spine up. Lift the hands and bend backward a little, pushing the hips a little outward. Tip to deepen this yoga stretch: Make sure that your biceps are next to your ears. The goal is to stretch up more rather than stretch backwards.

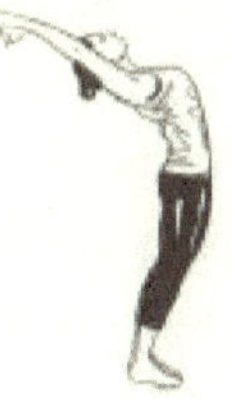

12. The Final Step - Pranāmāsana (Prayer pose):

Exhale and stand at the edge of your mat, keep your feet together and balance your weight equally on both feet. Open your chest and relax your shoulders. This finishes one round of Surya Namaskar.

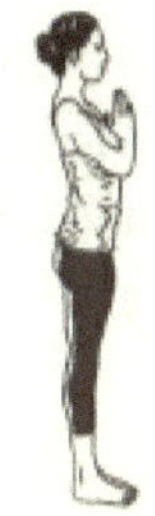

Siddhāsana (The Ultimate Way to Boost Your Vitality)

This is a secret method of the ancient sages. This seated yoga posture is superior to 84 other kinds of yoga. It is very helpful for celibacy and preserving the vital fluid. Imagine how a simple bike made of metal and rubber can take you on long journeys. That power is called "Kumbhak". Kumbhak means holding your breath for some time.

This seated yoga posture is called "Siddhāsana". It is the most potent and effective yoga because you can feel the positive effects very soon, but you need to eat simple and vegetarian food to get the best results.

How to do Siddhāsana?

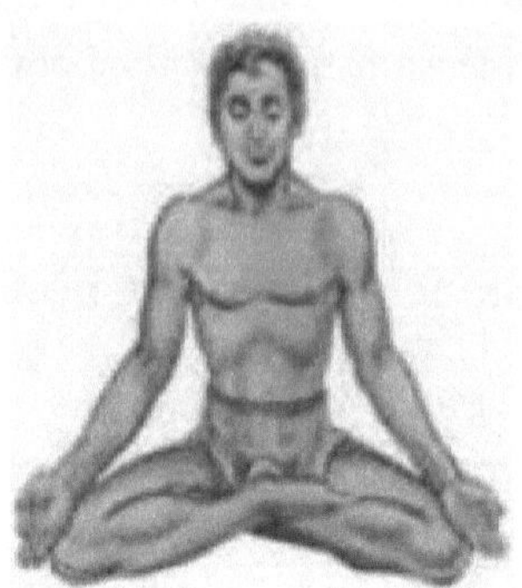

Do it on an empty stomach. Sit on a mat or a rug in a quiet place. Do Nādi Shodhan breathing exercise before or after this posture. Sit upright, and place your left heel near the area between your anus and your genitals. Place your right heel on your genitals. Breathe in deeply and try to hold it for one minute or as long as you can. This technique is different from triband; this breath retention is called Kumbhak; in this position, use positive affirmations. Do this for 2-3 rounds in a row. Whenever you feel negative about anything, do this right away, and you will see amazing results.

Benefits of Siddhāsana : It controls your sexual urges. It awakens your Kundalinī energy. It enhances your alertness and enthusiasm, heals nocturnal emissions and seminal disorders. It sharpens your mind. It cultivates noble qualities in life. It removes impurities and negative energy from your body. It creates positive thoughts to follow a good daily routine. It aids in meditation effortlessly.

Vajrāsana (A Simple and Powerful Sitting Yoga Posture):

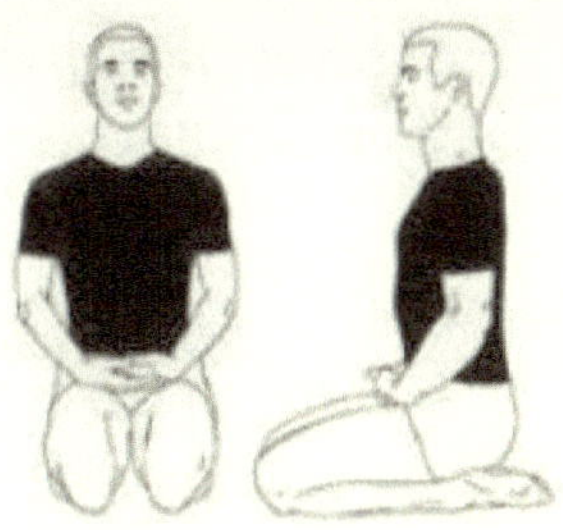

This is a basic sitting yoga posture that is named after the Sanskrit word vajra, which means diamond or thunderbolt. In this posture, you sit on your legs with your knees bent and your feet pointing backwards. This takes the pressure off your knees and allows you to do breathing and meditation exercises in this position, which can make your body as strong as a diamond.

Benefits of Vajrāsana: It aids in the digestion of food. It eases or avoids constipation. It fortifies the pelvic muscles.

Steps of Vajrāsana: Kneel down on the floor. You may use a yoga mat for comfort. Bring your knees and ankles close together and align your feet with your legs. The tops of your feet should face the floor with your big toes touching. Breathe out as you sit on your legs. Your hips will rest on your heels, and your calves will rest on your thighs. Place your hands on your thighs and tilt your pelvis slightly back and forth until comfortable. Breathe in and out slowly as you sit up tall by lengthening your spine. Use your head to lift your body up and push your tailbone down. Align your head to look forward with your chin parallel to the floor. Rest your hand palms down on your thighs with your arms relaxed.

The Magic of Pranayama

As I explained in the 13th rule of Brahmacharya, prāna is the vital energy that flows through our breath (Swās)in the human body. Prānāyāma is the practice of breathing more mindfully. When you cultivate the habit of conscious breathing, you will become more aware of yourself. This will help you to discern what your body needs and what can harm your Brahmacharya.

Practicing prānāyāma not only prevents the loss of Brahmacharya, but also helps to sustain it for a longer period. It gives you spiritual peace and mental fortitude to stay mentally super strong. Now I will introduce you to some prānāyāma techniques that can be very beneficial for your Brahmacharya journey.

Nādi Shodhan Prānāyāma

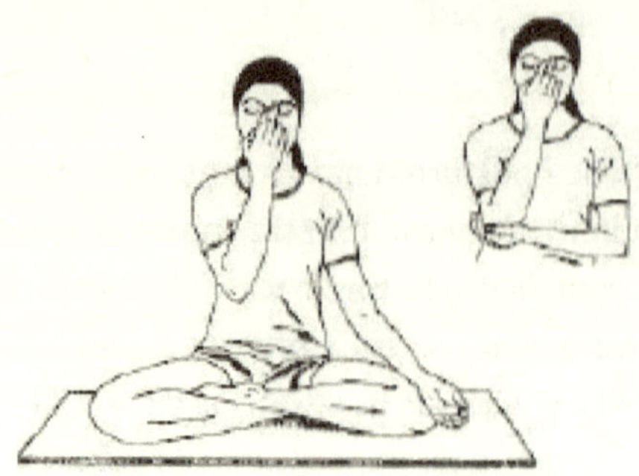

Nādi = subtle energy channel; Shodhan = cleaning, purification; ā= breathing technique. Nadis are subtle energy channels in the human body that can get clogged for various reasons. The Nadi Shodhan Prānāyāma is a breathing technique that helps to clear these obstructed energy channels, thus soothing the mind. This technique is also known as Anulom Vilom Prānāyāma. (**Note: x:y = 2:1**)

Method: Sit comfortably with your spine straight and shoulders relaxed. Keep a gentle smile on your face. Place your left hand on the left knee, and palms facing up or in Chin Mudra (thumb and index finger lightly touching at the tips). Place the tip of the right hand's index finger and middle finger between the eyebrows, the ring finger and little finger on the left nostril, and the thumb on the right nostril.

We will use the ring finger and little finger to open or close the left nostril and thumb for the right nostril. Press your thumb gently on the right nostril and breathe in slowly through the left nostril. Now hold your breath for x seconds. Now breathe out for y seconds from the right nostril and press the left nostril softly with the ring finger and little finger. Now inhale from the right nostril, and hold your breath for x seconds. Breathe out from the left nostril for y sec. You have now completed one round of Nadi Shodhan Prānāyāma.

Continue breathing in and out from alternate nostrils. Complete seven such rounds by switching between both nostrils.

After every exhalation, remember to breathe in from the same nostril from which you exhaled. Keep your eyes closed throughout, and continue taking long, deep, smooth breaths without strain or effort.

Benefits: This is an excellent breathing technique to calm and centre the mind. Our mind tends to dwell on the past or worry about the future. Nādi Shodhan Prānāyāma helps to bring the mind back to the present moment. Works therapeutically for most circulatory and respiratory problems. Releases accumulated stress in the mind and body effectively helps to relax. Most people ejaculate when they are stressed and find that, ultimately, they are increasing their stress. Nādi Shodhan Prānāyāma is a natural way to break this cycle. It helps to balance the left and right hemispheres of the brain, which correspond to the logical and emotional sides of our personality. It helps to cleanse and harmonise the nādis - the subtle energy channels, thereby ensuring a smooth flow of prāna (life force) throughout the body. Maintains body temperature.

Caution

1. Do not force your breathing; keep the flow gentle and natural. Do not breathe from the mouth or make any sound while breathing.

2. Place the fingers very lightly on the forehead and nose. There is no need to apply any pressure.

3. Maintain a gap of 2 hours before practicing this Prānāyāma.

Tribandh Prānāyāma

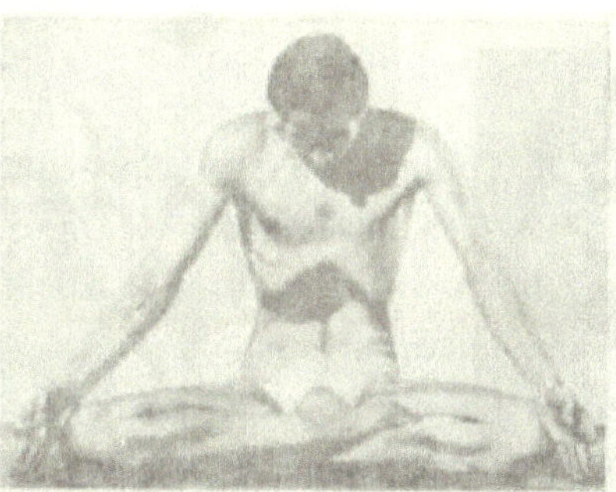

Tribandh Prānāyāma

Prāna, the ancient force that animates the universe, manifests in humans as breathing breath. One can gain control over the body and mind by regulating the breath. Tribandha, or '3 locks', are essential to Prānāyāma or breathe control.

Tribandha Prānāyāma involves these three Bandhas: *Jālandhara bandha*, *uddiyāna bandha*, and *mula bandha*. These bandhas strengthen glands, nerves, and cells, keeping the body fit and healthy.

Jālandhara Bandha (Chin Lock)

Jālandhar bandha was devised by māhasiddha yogi, Jālandhar, of the Nātha tradition, for focus and mental stability through breath retention. To do it, be in a comfortable position, resting your hands on the knees. Breathe in deeply and hold the breath, leaning the torso forward. Lower your head, and press the chin against the throat as much as possible. Bring attention to the ājnā chakra in the middle of the eyebrows, and breathe out after 10-15 seconds. Repeat the cycle five times or more.

Another method is to hold the breath outside and place the chin in the hollow of the throat. With the contraction of the throat and the closure of Idā and Pingalā nādis (energy channels starting from the lower abdomen below the navel and ending at the base of the forehead), the vishuddha chakra at the base of the throat is activated.

The secretion of nectar from brahmarandhra on top of the head is preserved; otherwise, it flows down to Manipura chakra, at the level of the navel, and is burned in the stomach fire.

Uddiyāna Bandha (Abdominal Lock)

'Uddiyana' means 'to fly up. Uddiyāna bandha helps to lift the obstructed Apāna Vāyu in the abdomen towards Sushumnā-Nādi, the central nerve channel running along the spine. Sit comfortably, keep your spine straight and inhale, expand your abdomen, and pull the abdomen inwards and up, combining it with breath. Repeat the exercise a few times. Uddiyāna bandha should be done on an empty stomach after emptying the bowels. It stimulates Manipura chakra, and it increases metabolic processes.

Mula Bandha (Root Lock)

When the three locks are applied together systematically, it is called maha bandha, a great lock. Mulabandha can be done by lifting the anus and urinary bladder upwards. It is best done in the lotus position and Bhaya Kumbhaka, where breath is held inside.

Alternatively, while sitting, one must press the perineum with the left heel and place the right heel over the genitals, followed by contraction of the pelvic floor muscles for 15-20 times. As a result, Apāna Vāyu, which naturally tends to move downwards, rises and merges with Prāna Vāyu at the heart centre. With practice, both Vayu-s join into Brahma nādi, 'just as a serpent enters its hole.' Brahma nādi (Sushumnā) is a subtle stream of kundalinī energy as it moves towards Sahasrāra at the crown of the head. Mulabandha balances Muladhara chakra at the base of the spine and makes a Yogi an Urdhvareta whose energy moves upwards.

Bhastrikā Prānāyāma

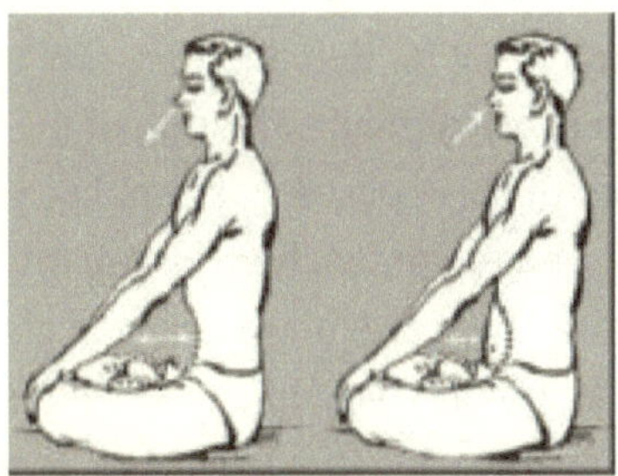

When we exercise, our body needs more oxygen, which makes the heart beat faster, thus increasing the heartbeat. But did you know that by doing Bhastrikā Prānāyāma, you supply more oxygen without the body demanding it?

Bhastrika Prānāyāma is the quick breathing in and out process which energises the body and is rightly called the yogic fire breath.

So, the next time you feel your body lacks energy, try BhastrikāPrānāyāma instead. Bhastrikā Prānāyāma is the most effective energy provider than other practices. Try it before meditation for better focus.

Method: Sit in vajrāsana or sukhāsana (cross-legged position). Make your body relaxed. (Prānāyāma can be more effective in Vajrayana as your spine is straight and the diaphragmatic movement is better.)

Put your hand on your lap. Bhastrikā prānāyāma is done in three speeds: slow, medium, and fast. Inhale and exhale with the same intensity (High Energy), starting this slowly and changing to a medium and fast pace. Do it 100 times at a slow speed and then increase the speed of breathing in and out to medium and then to fast speed and the counting up to 100 times. Practice increasing the number of rounds for better results.

Benefit: Great for revitalizing the body and mind. Since we use our lung capacity to the fullest while doing it, the prānāyāma helps eliminate toxins and impurities. It helps with sinus, bronchitis, and other respiratory issues. It enhances awareness and sensory acuity. It helps to balance doshas.

Yoga Nidra -Receiving Cosmic Energy

The way you sleep affects how much cosmic energy you receive. Yoga Nidra is a superior form of sleep that refreshes your tired mind and gives you more vitality after waking up. It draws cosmic energy for a higher level of spirituality even when you are asleep. The right way to sleep - Yoga Nidra was introduced by Paramhansa Yogānanda in 1936. He taught us how to tap into cosmic energy during sleep and use it in every difficult situation of life. Paramhansa Yogānanda explained the importance of this special posture. Let your internal organs rest in the bowl of your chest and abdomen. It gives you internal relaxation, and you can stay in this position for several nights as the Yogi claimed. He is so internally recharged that he can keep his eyes open and stay awake for many days. This is the power of cosmic energy. In ancient times, many yogis and yoddhas (great warriors) fought battles for many years without stopping. This shows how cosmic energy gives them the ability to do various tasks.

Relax your muscles and lie down in corpse posture; place both hands on your abdomen. Close your eyes and think, "I can stay in yoga nidra for several nights by closing my eyes' ' Hold for 20 seconds. After 20 seconds, open your eyes. Now think that you are energised by cosmic energy, raise your eyeballs and feel like "I am entering the state of superconscious bliss" All my organs are going to that state of relaxation. My heartbeat is now calm and relaxed.

After reaching a deep relaxation, I have attained superconscious bliss. Remain in this state, and you will naturally fall asleep by closing your eyes. This is Yoga Nidra. Hold for 20 seconds here.

Benefits of Yoga Nidra:

1. **Increase of Life Energy:** After getting cosmic energy, life energy is increased. Lifespan and health improve greatly. Ancient sages could live for several hundred years. In this modern age, Mahāvatār Bābāji is still alive in the Himalayas for 2000 years.

2. **Purifies your subconscious mind:** The person with a weak subconscious mind has many illusory thoughts and desires in his mind, and he is trapped in the cycle of false happiness, worries and pain. He cannot sleep well due to illusory dreams. The subconscious mind is cleansed by practicing Yoga Nidra which affects your thinking and action positively. The person feels energised after getting up from sleep.

3. **Free from Distraction:** No distraction will bother you because cosmic intelligence influences your intelligence. You gain tremendous self-control power. Your mind will be focused and centred easily.

4. **Nādi purification:** Purification of 72000 nādis or energy channels of our body. Negative attitude, stress or thought cause various problems in your energy channels followed by an increase of different diseases. But by practicing Yoga Nidra, you get cosmic energy which allows the life energy to flow smoothly through 72000 nādis without any obstacle. Your body will have an aurā that can be seen using advanced equipment.

5. **Internal organs rejuvenation:** The power and functions of the internal organs are enhanced by the influence of cosmic energy. It heals many internal diseases. It gives you tremendous life energy and deep relaxation of your internal organs. Yoga Nidra can be compared with a spiritual bath deep inside the nectarine ocean. There is no energy shortage, and your mind will not experience any restlessness or weakness rather lost in super consciousness state.

Techniques For Conquering Sexual Desire

In the pursuit of overcoming unwanted sexual desire, it's essential to adopt practical strategies that empower individuals to regain control over their minds. This chapter explores a variety of approaches, drawing inspiration from practices that have proven effective.

Begin by immersing yourself in the fresh air or engaging in brisk physical activity, such as strolling in fresh air, physical exercise, or running half to one mile to pacify the sexual desire. Contemplate the exemplary lives of the great men who have strictly adhered to Brahmacharya, finding inspiration from their commitment.

When Sexual Desire Attacks You Try The Following Remedies

1. Meditate on the great celibates in your heart. By remembering their sublime spiritual teachings, your sex impulse will be curbed.

2. Seek *satsang* or good company or engage yourself in talks with any great man on spiritual topics.

3. Read religious books so that your lust cannot trouble you.

4. When the sex desire arises, never stay in seclusion. If your sex desire is overpowering you, drink more cold water than you want.

5. Have a bath in cold water. If possible, take a rub and scrub bath in any river. Wash your head with cold water as long as your mind does not become steady.

6. Eat any sour fruit, even if you don't like it.

7. Massage your ears vigorously.

8. Do Bhastrika Pranayama (the bellow breathing) for 15-20 minutes.

9. Visualize the cremation ground or think about the burial or cremation of a dead body.

10. Think about the vanity of the world, and despise the perishable nature of your body.

11. The best way to overcome lust is to shift your focus away from sex to some creative activity that does not harm you.

12. Ponder over the mysteries of creation, dissolution, or reflect on personal experiences such as the loss of a loved one or past hardships, as these can aid in curbing sex desire.

13. Meditate on God and remember him constantly.

By practicing the abovementioned time-tested techniques, you can pacify sex desire.

Tantric Sex and Yoga Practices

I would like to draw an important conversation regarding Tantric sex from the book "*The Role of Celibacy in Spiritual life*" by Swami Chidananda.

Question: Tantra or the practice of "Sacred Sexuality," is becoming very popular in the West today. Do you think these teachings offer an authentic spiritual path?

Swamiji: No, I do not think that these teachings offer an authentic spiritual path. Why? Because of human frailty, human weakness. The human mind is so made that it always takes the easy way. Tantra is a way of reaching God through all kinds of sense enjoyment. Everything is offered to God and so everything becomes holy; nothing is impure. One enjoys sense satisfaction and sees it also as part of God's bliss. There is a view, and it has some merit, that while in all human experiences duality remains—there is an "I am enjoying this object" feeling—that in the ultimate sexual experience between a truly loving male, deeply in love with the female and fully reciprocated by the female, there is no awareness of one's separate individuality. [150]

There is a complete merging of the separatist consciousness in each one, and there is only the awareness of bliss experience. There is no personal identity remains who experiences. They say this is a possibility when it is done to its perfection. The two cease to be and there is only one, non-dual experience, absolute, Brahmic- consciousness. So they say that the human body is a tool that, if properly used, can bring about a rising above body consciousness. For one in a million it may work.

The pursuit of pleasure is part of the Western view of life—not the renunciation of pleasure. And one teacher in ten may be an authentic teacher genuinely offering something suited to the Western temperament. But nine of them are very clever people. They know there is a demand for this, and they are smart to it.

The approach is: You can have your cake and eat it too. They said they were practising tantra but it was only drinking, eating, and sex pleasure. It took them nowhere, but I suppose it took them where they wanted to go. So it was called by enlightened people of that time as the "corrupted path." Two paths then came into existence: the authentic path which was called the "right-hand path," and the corrupted path which was only after enjoyment. That was called the "left-hand path." As I told you, the sex force is sacred; sex is sacred. It is one of the most sacred of all things. But sacred sexuality is a wrong term. Once you get involved in sexuality, the sacredness is gone. That is due to man's weakness, frailty. Therefore, I am not going to be a supporter of it.

Swami Kripalvananda in his book *Illusion of Conjugal Sadhana* writes, many sadhakas have raised questions directly or indirectly regarding the topic of conjugal sadhana. As I have been leading research for two years in the fields of yoga and music, it is appropriate that I provide the answers to the sadhakas' questions.

A Difficult Stage of Yoga : There is only one yoga. It has two types- *Sakama* and *niskama*. Both have various categories and different spiritual achievements. Whether it is Niskama Jnana Yoga, Niskama Bhakti Yoga or Niskama Karma Yoga, all start from Kriya Yoga, which itself begins with an important distinct stage. As this is a difficult stage of yoga, it is very hard to become stable in it. The sadhaka who rises to this stage is tormented by a very strong sensual urge.

Whenever he sits for his dhyana (meditation) session, he experiences intense arousal of the sexual instinct. Here the guidance of a Guru who is a perfect yogi is an absolute necessity.

If proper guidance is not available to the sadhaka, he does not have the courage to continue with his sadhana. From here the two main types of yoga branch out. In the first branch, the sadhaka satisfies his sexual desires with his wife in the natural way without asking her to meditate. Then he asks her to take meditation initiation from his Guru and both perform meditation together and take each other's help when their sexual appetite is aroused.

The followers of the Vama sect perform group meditation. They fix a schedule and then take each other's help in satisfying their desire. The follower of the second sect does not take feminine help. He leaves his meditation room when his sexual desire is aroused. He resorts to several ways which intuitively occur to him, but he is faced with only failure. At this stage, only a perfect and accomplished Guru can give the right guidance. The serious sadhakas of the Jnana, Bhakti, or Yoga cults all believe that sexual desires decrease with their practice of meditation.

Actually they increase, and when this happens, the sadhaka loses his faith. He tries to understand the reasons for this, but he cannot come up with an answer with which he can reconcile himself. The cause of the arousal of sexual desire is that the sex center is also the center of yoga. The sexual fluid is the medium in both sex and yoga.

The sex urge causes the sexual fluid to descend through ejaculation, and yoga causes it to ascend through sublimation.

The desire which is aroused at this stage of meditation is described in Srimad Bhagavad Gita as not contrary to the dharma or the law of religion. Lord Krsna says: "I am the strength of the strong, devoid of desire and passion. In beings I am the desire which is not contrary to the law of Dharma, O King of Bharatas (Arjuna)". Just as nature dons a special type of beauty in the autumn, summer, and rainy seasons, so also it dons new appearances during different life cycles. At the time when saints and ascetics were predominant, two different paths were followed ordinary and special. In the ordinary path, people practiced ordinary celibacy and tried to lead the life of a Brahmachari (chaste- celibate).

The people who followed the special path practiced yoga and tried to achieve perfection by becoming Urdhvaretas and accomplished yogis. Only a brave and great ascetic gathered the courage to follow the special path. The ordinary ascetics were considered unfit to practice yoga. So much importance was given to celibacy that the practice of celibacy became the main aim in the life of all ascetics and there was no one who believed in the practice of conjugal yoga. Due to the calmness prevailing in the minds of people, the practice of celibacy became easy in that age.

In the middle ages, sacrifice and dispassion declined and the tendency for accumulation grew. Talks of spiritual achievements and miracles were common in the towns. Various groups, Tantrika and Yogika, and different methods of yoga were being formed. The once costly salvation had become very cheap. The conjugal practice of yoga began at the end of this age. This was the origin of the

Vama Marga (left-handed path). Lord Siva, who overcame sexual power and then turned Cupid to ashes, left the city for the forests, and the ashes of Cupid did not stay ashes but were changed into godliness and came to dwell in the towns where they were revered. Self-control and virtuousness were also abandoned and were replaced by indulgence and evil deeds.

The Vaidika religion diminished, being replaced by un-vaidika features. Truth was replaced by falsehood, honesty became dishonesty. Hypocrisy in the name of yoga gradually took India into its grip. Through meditation, the circulatory system is activated. This results in the activation of the organs which produce sexual fluid. The Apana vayu is dominant here. To stop the activities of Apana, Prana descends and blocks it. Apana draws the sexual fluid towards the genitals, and Prana stops it from going in the lower direction. Apana enlarges the Susumna and Prana shrinks it.

Solitary and Joint Meditation: When the sadhaka is in the perilous position mentioned above, he or she is drawn towards the opposite sex. At this point, it is very important that the sadhaka be guided by an experienced Guru. If salvation were possible with sexual intercourse, then it would be said that salvation is not for the ascetic sadhaka, but only for the worldly sadhaka. If this is the case, then the virtue of dispassion has no meaning. On the other hand, the Holy Scriptures prescribe that only the dispassionate sadhaka is qualified for the path of salvation.

The materialistic sadhaka is not qualified for this great path. There are thousands of examples in the Puranas citing cases where a certain ascetic is said to have practiced intense penance and deep meditation which resulted in the shaking of Indrasana (the throne of Lord Indra), making him (Indra) fear his own security. To end this insecurity, Lord Indra would send a very beautiful nymph to go down to earth, attract the attention of the ascetic concerned, and destroy his penance. The nymph would go and disturb the ascetic by heavenly music and dancing, thus breaking his samadhi (union with the Almighty) and leading him astray into the realm of sensuality.

If sexual intercourse led one to salvation, then the presence of the nymph would have been a blessing to the ascetic. But this is not the case; on the contrary, the appearance of the nymph turns out to be a curse. These citations prove that one should practice sadhana alone. Surrender means the state in which the independent Prana, which is completely free from the bonds of the mind during meditation, is allowed to perform actions through the medium of the body and organs without any obstructions.

The Prana vayu is one of the five elements existing in nature. Though it seems dynamic, it is static. The source that instills life into Prana vayu is Paramesvara (God). It is not proper to leave this state of surrender to God in order to seek the protection of the opposite sex, i. e. another person. In sexual intercourse, the mind becomes extrovert and the sensory organs become uncontrollable. In spite of all this, sadhakas - both male and female - say that they experience the vital power functioning forcefully when they have sex. This experience is a result of their involvement in sexual pleasures and is an illusion.

This gross observation is far from the truth. The force that they experience is not that of Prana but that of the mind. Yes, during meditation the Prana sometimes becomes powerful, but it is never distracted. It is always calm. In this condition, it is not present in the external organs. It flows in the nadis or in the internal bodily passages. When husband and wife perform meditation together, their minds naturally dwell on each other. Therefore they are very soon affected by the force of lust and become excited. As clothes are obstructive during meditation, usually only the genitals are covered by a minimum of clothing.

The limbs are revealed. This also is a cause of excitement. Thus the presence of someone of the opposite sex is undesirable and obstructive. Furthermore, during meditation, when desire is awakened in the male, it may not have awakened in the female and vice versa. Under these circumstances, he or she imposes himself or herself on the other, disrupting the other's meditation and making the other yield to his or her wishes. Along with this, the couple who practice meditation together make another mistake. When the sexual instinct is aroused while meditating alone, it fades in few moments. But before it fades, the sadhaka gets himself in a more excited state and leads his partner also into his path.

In the meditation sessions of Vama margis (followers of the left-handed path) where sadhakas of both sexes perform meditation nude, lust is the dominant feature, so participants are soon stirred by it. Moreover, free sex is prevalent in this path and so it is easy to come in contact with new people every time. People who engage in these practices are only looking for new contacts and free sex.

Thus the aim of meditation is lost and pleasure takes its place. These sadhakas argue that just as you need iron to cut iron, so also you can overcome lust with lust. The argument seems convincing, but it is not correct; it can be proved to be false. It is true that iron cuts iron, but only an iron with a sharp edge can do so. If the iron used for cutting is not sharp it is cannot be used as a cutting tool.

When one resorts to the help of the opposite sex in meditation, the independent Prana becomes dependent, and yoga is transformed into pleasure. The sadhaka should never forget that in sexual pleasure there is a merging of the male and female, while in yoga the union is that of sadhaka and the Lord Almighty. The support of siddhasana and mudras and pranayama helps the Apana to ascend and open the gateway of salvation and closes the path leading to downfall. Through sexual intercourse, the Apana becomes descendant and never opens the closed gateway leading to salvation. Due to the various yogika kriyas, the purification of the blood takes place.

What are the Obstacles and Remedies: Some people say, "By adopting siddhasana and mudras, the attraction and inclination towards the opposite sex increase. Under these circumstances, mental impurities increase also. If a renunciated couple practice yoga together they will speed up their progress". When during meditation the Svadhisthana chakra is lit by yogika fires, the sexual instinct becomes intense. The sadhaka has to sublimate this intense sexual feeling. In order to do this, he or she should not seek the opposite sex.

If it had been possible to sublimate one's sexual feelings with the help of the opposite sex, then this whole world would have been the ideal place for penance and all householders would have become Urdhvareta saints. During meditation, control over the genitals is achieved by the practice of siddhasana and mudras which make Apana move upwards. In sexual intercourse, neither siddhasana nor the important mudras appear. As a result, there is no control over Apana and thus only pleasure is gained and not liberation. As the genital region becomes very sensitive during meditation, the sadhaka's mind becomes full of lustful thoughts. This inevitable situation must be patiently endured.

Lord Krishna mentions this stage of meditation: "Arjuna ! Even though one strives to practice yoga and is ever so discerning, his senses lead his mind away by force". The sadhaka watches as a witness the various actions performed by Prana during meditation. In the same way, he should also watch the wicked sensuous wanderings of the mind. The Muladhara chakra and the Svadhisthana chakra are related to each other. The Apana vayu rules these two regions. There is a collection of 72,000 nadis (bodily passages) in the legion of the Apana vayu.

Without the help of the kundalini, the purification of these nadis is not possible, to achieve the purification of these nadis is like crossing the Vaitarani River, a river which is said in the Puranas to be situated betweea Mrtyuloka (earth) and Yamaloka (the other world). It is full of very hot blood, bones, hair, etc. Sinners flounder in this river, unable to swim across it. Holy people swim across it by holding on to a cow's tail. Yogis consider the body, filled with blood, bones and hair, as the Vaitarani River. They use the cow's tail in the form of Kundalini to cross the river and become immortal.

It is better to die once while living with a smiling face than to die thousands of times crying and unwilling. To die a living death means to surrender oneself to God and to sacrifice oneself at his lotus feet. After the achievement of vajroli mudra, the sexual fluid of the sadhaka is not destroyed, and so he or she can become an urdhvareta and achieve a divine body, divine consciousness and complete detachment.

In India even today there are a few secret sects of Shiva, Vaisnava, and Shakti cults where men and women practice meditation together and try to achieve perfection in yoga. This path is called Vama marga (left handed path). It only spreads lust, and the generation which follows becomes dull and uncultured. Self-restraint and limited companionship of women or men should hold a place of primary importance in the practice of yoga for the ordinary person. The more restraint one practices, the more spiritual power he attains. With this power, he achieves wealth, spouse, children, fame, and other material achievements. He must find ways to conserve his sexual fluid. If a householder receives *shaktipata* (Transfer of energy from a Guru to a disciple) and practices it zealously, he becomes scattered, unrestrained, and talkative. As a result, he fails in the eyes of society and becomes frustrated.

Warning Experience Of A Tantric Meditator : A tantra practitioner named Hugh Milne who was a loyal follower of famous Osho cult, revealed how uncontrolled sex with the practice of tantra taught in the book "From Sex To Superconsciousness" can lead to severe mental disorders, insanity, STDs, and even death. In his book "Bhagwan - The God that failed". He shared his experience as follows.

I was released from the hospital after a week, but I was still on Valium. I was in a state of deep despair. I had lost all the happiness and fun in my life, and I felt that I was destined to fail forever. I recalled the early days with Bhagwan as a glorious time that would never come back. While I was in this risky state of mind

I attempted to end my life. I consulted a London psychiatrist, who suggested that the best thing for me was to return to the ranch. I was horrified by his evaluation. I stayed three more weeks in psychiatric hospital, believing at first that I would never get out.

At the Festival in 1984, Sheela announced that three sannyasis had succumbed to AIDS, though they were not identified. Sheela recommended to Bhagwan that condoms and rubber gloves should be used to prevent the transmission of the virus. He agreed, along with some rules meant to limit sexual activity among his disciples. What a contrast from the exciting days of Bombay when he had declared that sex was sacred!

When Krishnamurti labeled Bhagwan a criminal, I think he was not talking about the violation of legal laws. He was talking about his abuse of hypnosis and psychic powers. Perhaps the most evident of the psychic connections that sannyasis had with Bhagwan was their mala, and it was not surprising to learn that when sannyasis received their mala at darshan, they were instructed that if they ever took it off they should give it back personally to Bhagwan.[151]

What we can learn from this story is the dark side of Trantric teachings and practices. Hugh Milne has exposed saying Osho manipulated his followers with hypnosis and psychic powers, and how his philosophy of sex and tantra led to physical and mental harms. He also revealed the hypocrisy and corruption of Osho's inner circle, and the crimes they committed in the name of enlightenment. This chapter is a warning to those who are tempted by the allure of the charisma of any such Tantric Guru and its promises, and a reminder that not everything that glitters is gold.

CHAPTER XXV

What And How to Eat for Brahmacharya

As we have already explained, eating unhealthy food will not make you healthy. Many people settle for less nutritious food because they think it is expensive and difficult to prepare and store. However, the medical bills from poor health are much higher than the cost of healthy food. In this chapter, we will discuss the ideal food choices for a Brahmacharī or anyone who wants to live a healthy life.

Nutritious Breakfast:

1. **How to eat Raisins (Kishmish):** Raisins should be washed thoroughly before eating, as they may have dust and impurities on them. Rinse them at least 1-2 times and you will see the water becoming dirty. After washing them well, place them on a clean cloth and let them dry. Mix the following ingredients in the specified quantities: 20-25 Raisins, 5 Almonds, 10 Peanuts, one bowl of sprouted Moth beans, one bowl of Nuts, and one bowl of Moong beans in a Large Bowl. Fill this bowl with water and leave it overnight. Remember, you have to soak the raisins in a separate bowl. In the morning, drain the water from both bowls, but do not discard the water from the raisin bowl. This water is very rich in nutrients and good for drinking. It also helps to improve the skin and complexion. Now combine all six ingredients and eat them as breakfast. The amount suggested in this recipe is suitable for your intake, not too little or too much.

2. **Moth Bean Breakfast:** Moth beans are one of the simplest and most nutritious breakfasts. However, not many people know how to eat them properly. If you follow the recommended method, you will get the best results.

The correct method is: First, wash them with water in a bowl, then soak them in a bowl full of water for 3-4 hours. Next, drain the water from the moth beans and spread them on a clean cloth. Then, wrap the beans in the cloth, making a pouch of beans. Leave them overnight. In the morning, you will see that the beans have sprouted. You can eat them without salt, which is the best option, or you can add a little salt if you prefer.

Tips for Increasing Vital Fluids in the Body

1. **Using Limestone:** Calcium deficiency is very common among young boys and girls. This causes two major problems for the body. First, the bones become weak and second, the sperm count decreases. Limestone is a good source of calcium, which can remedy both of these problems. However, you should use it in moderation, not in random amounts. You should take a piece of limestone as small as a wheat grain and dissolve it in a spoon of water. You can add this water to a bowl of curd, any vegetable curry, or even any juice. This practice can greatly enhance the strength of your bones and increase your sperm count.

2. **Using Jaggery:** You should eat a piece of jaggery as big as a lemon after breakfast or dinner. Jaggery has many benefits, but here are some of them: it boosts your digestion power, it increases your blood production and circulation.

3. **Eating Āmlā (Indian gooseberry):** Āmlā is very good for blood purification and cleansing of Muladhara Chakra. You should eat one or two Āmlās daily for better skin tone, facial glow, and other benefits related to skin and blood circulation.

One ultimate Homemade remedy for all sexual problems:

Men and women in this era are frustrated with their health and low vitality. Men face the problem of semen leakage during urination or sometimes even by slight excitement. Women face the problem of white discharge. You can solve all these problems by using this solution.

Combine 250 gm of Triphala Powder, 250 ml of Black Sesame Oil, and 250 ml of Pure Honey and keep it in a glass jar. Take 10 gm of this mixture in the morning and another 10 gm at night. After consuming this, you should drink one glass of warm water. This can boost your vitality and provide all the necessary nutrients for your body. You will notice the change in just one month of using this, and in 3 months, you will recover all the vitality you have lost due to improper habits.

Eating habits:

I advise you to avoid eating food late at night. When you eat food, it begins to digest in your body, generating heat in the process. Humans are not designed to cope with this heat, and this can lead to losing Brahmacharya due to the heat from digestion. Let me elaborate on this. Digestion is a process that releases heat. The body emits this heat naturally, but this heat can have two effects. One, it disrupts the sleep cycle of the human body and stimulates the body to release heat, which can indirectly cause nightfall and other forms of semen loss. I recommend everyone to be disciplined about the timing of food. Try to have your dinner before 7PM or you can skip your dinner whenever possible.

Exercise for Sublimation of Vital Energy

Your vitality depends on your diet, thoughts, and lifestyle. We will explore the lifestyle guidelines given by the ancient and modern sages. Semen is the essential vital energy, and we will reveal the secret of how to live in a way that preserves your vital energy. This tip is guaranteed to work. It will help you achieve a vibrant life, which is the only meaningful way to live.

Method: You have to run in place. Keep your chest up. You have to run on your toes. Your heels should not touch the floor, and your feet should not make noise. Bring your foot to your buttocks one at a time. Stay in the same spot while running. Start this exercise slowly, and then speed up.

Warning: People with heart problems should do it gently.

Why this Exercise is good for you:

This exercise eliminates lethargy completely. It makes you more energetic. It fortifies your heart and lungs and keeps them healthy. It allows semen to rise up. Your life energy (sexual energy) moves to higher levels where it becomes Ojas. It cleans your intestines and improves your appetite. Wet dreams will stop after one month, and many other illnesses will be cured.

How to retain more vital energy:

Many people overeat tasty food, which is very bad for them. Eat less than you feel hungry if you are fit or overweight. Try to eat in a nice place when your mind is calm and happy. Do not fill your stomach at night. It puts pressure on your body organs which can cause serious diseases. It is also a cause of wet dreams. Eat light food at night. Chew your food well, and do not drink water before eating. Drink water after 45-60 minutes of eating. Eating after midnight is not healthy for you. A person who has problems with wet dreams should not drink milk at night before sleeping. Spinach, green leafy vegetables, milk, butter, ghee, buttermilk, ripe fresh fruits, and white pumpkin are pure foods that help you maintain Brahmacharya. They also make your thinking positive.

Fasting every two weeks on Ekadashi is good for your digestion and helps you overcome normal thoughts of sex and anger. Wet dreams usually happen in the last part of the night. So, get out of bed between 4 and 4:30 AM. Those who wake up early in the morning become spiritual easily. Alcohol, cigarettes, and tobacco affect your emotions. By using drugs, your lungs and heart become weak, your stamina decreases, and your life energy reduces. Your aging process speeds up. Your semen becomes watery because of toxins. Always be happy. Do not dwell on the past and always feel energy in your mind. There is no power greater than your mental power. Improve yourself in the present.

CHAPTER XXVI

Debunking The Misconceptions About Brahmacharya

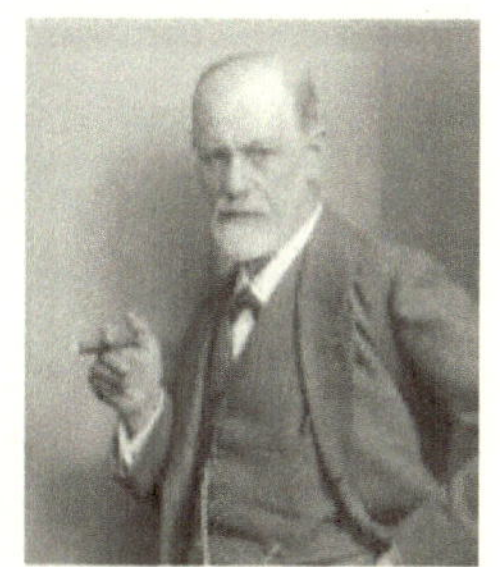

Sigmund Freud, the founder of psychoanalysis, thought that sexual urges and hidden sexual feelings were very important for human behaviour. He thought that sexual energy, or libido, was the main motivation for human behaviour and influenced all human thinking and action.

Sigmund Freud had many unresolved sexual issues with himself. His idea of constitutional bisexuality, for example, was a rationalization for some of his personality traits. I think many analysts are smart and committed people, but analysis tends to draw those with a personality like Freud's—passive men and aggressive women." This boldly expressed doubt about the leader would usually be confined to bathroom talk at neo-Freudian meetings. But it was said during an interview with Dr. Harold M. Voth, a psychiatrist who teaches at the Menninger Foundation and a member of The American Psychoanalytic Association. Dr. Voth believes that Freud showed "a significant amount of femininity" in his personality, a trait that has affected the whole profession by making what he calls "neurotically troubled" Dr. Freud a model.

The personality of Sigmund Freud, who died almost forty years ago, lives on in the fields of psychotherapy, psychoanalysis, and much of modern psychiatry. Freud's personal wants and conflicts have become almost indistinguishable from the entire structure of the Psychological Society that he created.

Freud used cocaine on and off for almost fifteen years. At first he used it for emotional reasons, but later the cocaine was a nose treatment for his sinusitis, a therapy suggested by Dr. Fliess, who was a nose doctor. (Breathing in through the nose is a common way of getting "high" on cocaine.) During the 1890s, Dr. Max Schur tells us, Freud used "frequent local applications of cocaine." No one has yet assessed the hallucinatory effect of cocaine on Freud's mind during the early years of psychoanalysis. Without cocaine, could Freud have invented such unlikely fantasies of human imagination? The cocaine episode was one of the many unscientific adventures of the Vienna nerve doctor-turned-philosopher.

Freud's sexual toxicological theory—that the body could be poisoned by sexual dissatisfaction—was another scientific mistake that became part of popular belief. The lack of enough sexual activity blocked the libido and caused chemical substances that harmed the mind, he theorized. Freud said that the physical effect of this process caused the "actual neurosis" (the German word was aktuell, or current) while its mental effect was a psychoneurosis.

He split the patients into two groups, those suffering from either anxiety neurosis or neurasthenia. Anxiety neurosis was caused by the frustration of "coitus interruptus, unfulfilled arousal and sexual abstinence." In neurasthenia it was sexual abuse: "too much masturbation and too many wet dreams." The remedy was simple: more sex. "If it was possible to stop the abuse and replace it with normal sexual activity, a remarkable improvement in the condition was the result," Freud promises us.

The theory has now been abandoned, but Freud's childish idea of a body poisoned by sexual dissatisfaction continues in common psychological belief. The Oedipal love triangle is a main example of how Freud's personality has twisted psychology and psychiatry.

During his self-analysis, Freud found out that he felt love for his mother and envy against his father. As an adult, he had a repeated thought in which he pictured his "beautiful and thin" mother, Amalie.

Based on his belief in the trauma of the primal scene (watching one's parents during sex), Freud as a boy must have seen his attractive mother having sex. What might have been ignored by a less obsessed child seemed to control Freud.

Freud clearly felt oedipal desire, a problem that non-Freudians, such as child psychiatrist Dr. Stella Chess of New York University, think only affects a few children. He then had the illusion that his abnormality was normal and universal. "With boys the wish to have a child with their mother is always there," he wrote. Ernest Jones has named this single-idea fixation, which made Freud extend his own feelings to all people, as both Freud's great strength and his crippling weakness. In the case of the oedipal theory, Freud has imposed his own sick childhood on modern society as a usual situation, thus making psychic disorder in the Psychological Society.

As a young boy, young Sigmund showed strange behavior. At the age of seven he went into his parents' bedroom and purposely peed on the floor. He called himself a sufferer of neurasthenia, a term that included modern neuroticism and a kind of hypochondria. Freud said he had "a mild case of typhoid," and "a light case of smallpox" when he was young. Dr. Schur has shown that many simple stomach diseases were then called "mild typhoid." Once, after staying in bed for "sciatica," he decided "not to have sciatica anymore" and just got up. One odd neurotic sign was his habit of fainting.

He was known to have fainted at least four or five times. Once it was because of seeing bleeding blood. Usually it was because of some insult to his huge ego. In 1909, just before they went to America, Freud and Jung were in Bremen. Freud told his follower that he, Jung, had hidden death wishes against him. Jung strongly denied it. During the fight Freud suddenly fainted. . , In 1912 Freud and Jung argued again over an article in which Jung had not mentioned Freud. Jung was sorry, but Freud kept on criticizing, then suddenly dropped to the floor in a faint. Jung took him to a sofa.

Freud's first words when he woke up were: "How nice it must be to die." Modern psychoanalysis, much of modern psychiatry and most of psychotherapy are the exact reflections of those neuroses.

They are the caring home for Freud's deadly death wishes, disastrous sibling conflicts, hidden hatred against parents, bisexuality, incest urges, hidden homosexuality, reversed love-hate feelings, dogmatic beliefs and invisible hates of every kind. ' It is a unique victory. It is the transfer of one man's anger into a whole culture. Children do not usually or even often hate new children in the family. Nor are most people hidden homosexuals or unconscious bisexuals. Nor do most boys secretly wish their fathers dead as Freud did. Nor is the childish sex experience the cause of our personality. Nor is mixed love-hate the norm for most emotions.

We should ask one question. What if Freud had not had a tight colon, constant sad moods, neurasthenia, homosexual feelings, bad mood, headaches, constipation, travel fears, death fears, heart problems, money fears, infected noses, fainting fits and aggressive feelings of hate and murder? Would the modern theory of the mind have been more positive? Would it have instead emphasized the sympathy and care that people have for their siblings, their parents, even for all people? What if Freud had not been a victim of belief, magic numbers and childish naivety? Would psychiatry and psychotherapy today show the influence of a more scientific and logical approach to the human mind?

The Freudian sickness has penetrated our minds and our society more than we realize. If we see that a lot of it is a mirror of Freud himself, and we understand the extent of that personality flaw, it may help us to escape from its widespread impact. We may not have to live under the dark cloud of Dr. Freud.[152]

We saw Freud did not use two well-known scientific methods to back up his ideas. He rejected using clinical trials with experimental and control groups to see if his therapy worked. He also did not think it was important to observe and study children to support his ideas about how they grow. Now, let's look at what he thought about the third major method scientist's use - experiments where you change one thing and see how it affects another thing.

Freud's opinion on experiments, the most important scientific method, is clear in a postcard to Rosenzweig in 1934. Rosenzweig told him how he tried to study repression through experiments. Freud said, 'I don't care much about these confirmations because I already have many reliable observations that support my ideas, making them independent of experiments.' He politely added, 'Still, it doesn't hurt.' This shows Freud did not think experiments were needed to prove or change his ideas. No other field has completely closed itself off from experimental testing, not even astrology or phrenology.

To quote T.H. Huxley, who talked about the tragedy of science - killing a beautiful theory with an ugly fact. Freud tried to protect his theory by making it hard to test. Even after 80 years, there is still no strong experimental evidence, clinical studies, statistics, or observations supporting Freudian theories. As Michael Faraday said, 'They reason theoretically without demonstrating experimentally, and errors are the result.' These words might be suitable for the end of psychoanalysis as a scientific idea.

Psychoanalysis is at best an early and false set of ideas. At worst, it's a pseudo-scientific belief that has harmed psychology and psychiatry and let down many patients who believed in it. It's time to see it as a history thing and focus on building a truly scientific psychology.

Freud's criticisms extend to his followers like Jung and Adler. Most of them moved away from scientific rigor, like Jung, who turned to mysticism. I won't talk much about those who rebelled against Freud, but Jung, Melanie Klein, Wilhelm Stekel, Alfred Adler, and many others belong to that list.

Some psychologists, like Carl Jung, disagreed with Freud on concepts like the unconscious mind and libido. Alfred Adler proposed his theory focusing on social factors and the drive for superiority. Karen Horney criticized Freud's emphasis on sexual instincts, suggesting social and cultural factors shape personality more. Erik Erikson expanded on Freud's stages by adding psychosocial influences. Behaviorists like B.F. Skinner and John B. Watson rejected Freud's focus on the unconscious mind, concentrating on observable behavior and the environment.

Freud's interest in sexual sublimation, oedipal rivalry, and penis envy might have been driven by personal concerns. In his dreams, he felt emasculated, deprived of sexual rights by his wife, and that his children turned his sexual organs into relics. According to Carl Jung, Freud's one-time friend, he got involved with his sister-in-law Minna during this time. Jung's American disciple, John Billinsky, shared this story, quoting Jung's surprise and agony at learning about Freud's intimate relationship with Minna. Jung, despite his own extra-marital relations, found Freud's situation shocking.[153]

You need to realize that modern science will take a long time to comprehend the true meaning of sexual energy and discover the power of Brahmacharya, but the Vedic science has already revealed the benefits of semen retention and Brahmacharya thousands of years ago. The impact of Brahmacharya on your mental health has been already described in many Hindu Scriptures. All myths about Brahmacharya are baseless. Please do not trust them. Reflect on practical theories of Veda, Scriptures, and Science and Opinions of Celibate scholars and follow the paths that lead to a specific eternal goal of life.

CHAPTER XXVII

Women And Brahmacharya

A seeker asks: "Does the same explanation of how Vīrya is formed and lost apply to women as well? Do they suffer the same consequences as men?" This is a relevant and important question. Indeed, sexual activity drains the female system and the male vitality.

It also puts a lot of stress on the system. The ovaries, the female organs that produce a substance like Vīrya, similar to the male testes, create, grow and mature a vital force called the ovum. Unlike men, who lose this force out of their body, women retain it inside. However, when they engage in sex, the ovum leaves the ovaries and is used to create the embryo. Childbearing is very exhausting and demanding for women. Losing this force repeatedly and going through childbirth ruin the health of women and damage their strength, beauty, grace, youth, and mental power. Their eyes lose the brightness and sparkle that show their inner forces. The strong sensual stimulation of the act damages the nervous system and causes weakness too. Women have a more sensitive and fragile system, so they are often more affected than men.

Women should protect their precious vitality. The ovum and the hormones that the ovaries secrete are crucial for women's optimal physical and mental well-being. It is obvious that reproduction is expensive for a female. They need special food when they are pregnant and breastfeeding, which shows that there is a cost involved. The female cost of reproduction is easy to understand because most of it happens at certain times, like pregnancy and breastfeeding. Also, a female stops being able to reproduce after a certain age. Their reproductive pattern means that they use up their body during short periods of stress and then stop completely after some time. Compared to this, a male human being can keep reproducing until he dies, which means that the costs are spread out more evenly throughout his life, and not so noticeable at any specific time. It is well known that a woman lives longer than a man in every country and situation. Many people think that this is because men have more testosterone. I personally think that this is because a woman stops being sexually fertile at middle age.

The menopause might give them the rest that they need after a busy sexual life. The men, on the other hand, are careless and keep draining themselves until the end, which makes them live shorter.

To show the female reproductive costs, I will mention an experiment where the bones of breastfeeding mothers who did not have enough calcium in their body lost calcium (Specker, 1994),[154] so that the milk could get the calcium it needs from the bones! This is shocking, but is it really? The female body would sacrifice its own health so that the baby does not go hungry. This experiment shows that the female's main goal is not her own long life, but her children's. We must therefore say that the costs of reproduction are as important for the female as they are for the male.[155]

A woman's sex life can impact her personality and how she carries herself even more than it does for a man. Being involved with many partners can toughen a woman, showing in her expressions and how she talks. It takes away from her natural gentleness, making her seem less soft and caring. On the flip side, when a man engages in too much sexual activity, it depletes his physical resources, while in women, it drains the nervous system and can lead to nerve issues or neurasthenia.

Having a lot of sexual encounters, more than anything else, can age a woman, sometimes even faster than it does for a man. It's widely known that intense romantic work, like what prostitutes do, speeds up aging. Excessive sexual activity and having different partners can affect a woman's vaginal and perineal muscles, leaving them weak, ineffective, and less sensitive.

Now, women have to deal with the biological outcomes of sexual relationships, mainly, the possibility of getting pregnant. The safest and surefire way to prevent pregnancy is by abstaining from sexual activities. It's completely safe, certain to work, and it's natural, with no side effects. Plus, it's available for free, no prescription needed for anyone. There's no artificial method of preventing pregnancy that offers all these benefits. The most effective artificial methods also come with serious, harmful side effects for women.

According to a two-page ad in a top medical journal mainly read by doctors, a popular birth control pill needs a whole page to list all the warnings, contraindications, precautions, and adverse reactions, including things like blood clots, liver issues, and even death. And, there's an adverse reaction that isn't listed – death. Engaging in sexual activities too often increases a woman's risk of getting cervical cancer. Also, starting romantic relationships too early in life raises the chances of getting cervical cancer. It's essential to be wise about these things.[156]

CHAPTER XXVIII

Brahmacharya After Marriage

According to Sanātana dharma, marriage is a sacred relationship between two souls, not just at the physical level but also at the spiritual level. It is not a license to indulge in sex whenever you feel like it. It is a connection of two souls in the presence of all family members, gods, stars, and the universe. That is why we worship God before getting married. In Sanātana Culture, there are some rules that should be followed to have a happy married life; if one follows all these rules, they will be regarded as Brahmachari even after marriage.

It may seem difficult to understand how to maintain Brahmacharya in marriage and enjoy your married life. First of all, what is the true meaning of Brahmacharya? Brahmacharya is a way of living with discipline, Spirituality, and Dharma. You must preserve your semen and keep your mind free from lust (Kāma). These are the basic rules for Brahmacharya and other rules are explained in Chapter 24. Now let's see how to practice Brahmacharya in the Grihastha āshram or householder life.

1. You may think that having no sex drive while married may harm your relationship. But that is not always the case. Marriage is not just a physical union of two opposite sexes but also a spiritual union of two souls. Marriage is a mutual support for each other to fulfill family and social duties, being one in every aspect of life whether it is love, success, failure, sorrow or happiness. Brahmacharya enhances married life and vice versa as it is related to the spiritual growth of the couple.

2. Anyone who wants to keep their marriage authentic and joyful has to practice Brahmacharya together. Otherwise, these sex drives and senses will ruin your non-sexual enjoyment. Couples who only have sex for fun or pleasure will never experience real love and the beauty of the Human body.

3. Sexual force is a creation of nature to sustain the race. Therefore, many scriptures have discussed the pros and cons of sexual energy. Living a continent life even after marriage is not hard if the couple follow a

spiritual lifestyle and listen to the teachings of great spiritual Gurus and Saints. Many spiritual Gurus and scriptures have clarified that Sexual force is given only for procreation. If we use it as a means of only sensual enjoyment, we are doing nothing but depleting our spiritual reservoir of life. Couples should manage how they will keep their life more spiritual and Vedic by avoiding sexual enjoyment as the core of their love life. This management will be challenging for one who is more lustful, but once you establish this management. You will never be lustful for your whole married life.

Couples who practice Brahmacharya have the best mental and Spiritual state. When they conceive, their spiritual power is transferred to their child. This child is born with the best of semen and ovum. This is why it is advised to conceive a child after having some time in the Brahmacharya state for both to beget intelligent, robust and talented children.

These are some Guidelines for (Grihasta) Householder by wise Spiritual Gurus:

1. A man should respect all women as mothers except his wife and never think of having contact with other women.

2. Strict control of sexual life and a firm practice of non-violence are essential if you want to advance on the spiritual path.

3. If you use contraceptives, you will never learn to practice self-restraint. He who uses contraceptives is an unethical man. Learn the virtue of self-restraint. The use of these unnatural methods will gradually drain your energy. It will destroy all restraints.

4. There is a close link between sex and control of the palate. He who has controlled the palate has already controlled all the other organs.

5. Sāttvic food will make the practice of Brahmacharya easy.

6. Continence is not harmful. On the contrary, it preserves nervous energy. It gives great mental strength and peace of mind.

7. Sexual indulgence leads to moral and spiritual ruin, early death, nervous weakness, and loss of one's faculties, talents, and abilities.

8. Manu says: *"The first-born child is born of Dharma and the rest of Kama or lust"*. The sexual act for mere pleasure is not acceptable". Passion for the flesh or body is not pure or real love. It is only attraction born of ignorance. You do evil deeds and kill your soul because of this passion.

If someone chooses not to get married right away and only has children sometimes for the sake of having a family, they can bring about kids who are healthy, smart, strong, attractive, and ready to make sacrifices. Long ago in India, wise and holy people, when married, followed this great rule, carefully. They taught others, through both actions and words, how to lead a disciplined life even while being married. Our ancestors indeed followed these wise individuals in creating families to protect their homeland and for other noble deeds. If you've read Srimad Bhagavata, you know about Devahuti, Manu's daughter, and her husband Kardama Rishi. Kapila Muni, the founder of the Sankhya philosophy, was born to Devahuti after Kardama Rishi visited her once to give her a son. Parasara visited Matsyagandha to bring forth Sri Vyasa, the founder of the Vedanta philosophy.

The great sages of the past were married, but they didn't live a life consumed by passion and desire. Their married life was centered on righteousness. If you can't exactly copy them, at least use their lives as guides, as an example to follow, and walk the path of truth. Married life isn't about indulging in desire and careless living. It's a disciplined life of selfless service, pure and simple righteousness, generosity, kindness, self-improvement, and everything good and helpful to humanity. If you can live such a life, being married is as good as living like a monk.

Live a well-balanced, moderate married life. Even as a married person, you can be disciplined, following the principles of marital duty, practicing moderation, and regularly worshiping God. Marriage shouldn't lead you away from your spiritual journey. Keep the spiritual flame burning. Help your wife understand the true glory of a spiritual life. If both of you practice self-discipline for a while and avoid excesses, she will give birth to strong children who will be a source of pride for the country. Conserving energy can be used for higher spiritual purposes.

Avoiding frequent pregnancies will also maintain your wife's health. Being disciplined in marital life means having moderate sexual relations. Married individuals are allowed to be together once a month at the right time, not for pleasure, but to have children and continue the family line. This too is a form of disciplined living. They are also practicing celibacy. Married individuals should encourage their wives to observe fasts and engage in practices like Japa, meditation, and others, which will help them maintain celibacy. Train your wives in studying the Gita, the Upanishads, the Bhagavata, and the Ramayana, and in regulating their diet.

If you want to practice celibacy, think of your wife as your sister. Remove the idea of husband and wife and cultivate the idea of brother and sister. This will create pure and strong love, free from the impurity of lust. Always talk to your wife about spiritual matters. Share stories from the Mahabharata, the Bhagavata. Spend time together on holidays reading religious books. Gradually, her mindset will change. She will take interest and find joy in spiritual practices. Put this into action if you want to escape the troubles of life and experience the eternal joy of the soul.

In today's world, many guys copy Westerners by always bringing their wives along when they go out. This makes them used to having women around all the time. Even a short separation can be really painful. Losing their wives can be a big shock, and it's tough for them to decide not to get married for even a month. That's pretty tough! Try spending less time with your life partners. Keep conversations short. Be serious. Don't laugh or joke too much. Take a walk in the evening. What did your smart ancestors do? Only adopt the good things from the West. Copying their fashion, style, clothes, and food is not a good idea.

CHAPTER XXIX

My Tips of Overcoming Adversity

This chapter is very dear to me, as it reflects the core message of this book. I will share with you how my morning meditation routine and the practice of Brahmacharya have transformed my life. I have already mentioned my first life changing book – *Divine Inspiration The Secret of Eternal Youth (Divya Prernā Prakāsh)* that rescued me from the path of ruin and instilled in me the sublime Sanskāra of Brahmacharya Lifestyle. This book was instrumental in helping me correct my chaotic lifestyle and improve it. I am grateful to God and the author and promoter of this book, which was a blessing for me. Here is my lifestyle routine when I was serving in the Indian Navy. However, I started doing Surya Namaskār only after I retired from the Naval service. The tips and routine that I have shared below are suitable for beginners. I have advanced my lifestyle to a higher level, which I have not included in this book.

The first thing I do every morning is Surya-Namaskār. I never miss it.

What are the benefits of doing Surya-Namaskār?

I have already explained the benefits of Surya-Namaskar earlier in this book. Please refer to that again, but I would like to highlight two amazing benefits that I have personally experienced. Firstly, if you do Surya-Namaskār every morning in front of the sun, you will look much younger. For example, if you are 40 or 45, you will look 10-15 years younger than your age. This is the miracle of Surya-Namaskār. You will also stay healthy and avoid getting sick easily. The second thing that I have personally experienced is that after doing Surya-Namaskār, meditation becomes very easy immediately. Your mind will quickly enter into a meditative state. Currently, I do 12 rounds of Surya Namaskār. You should also do at least 12 rounds. Some people do 20-30-50 rounds depending on their ability.

My second rule is fasting on Ekadashi day. Ekadashi comes every 15 days. I will tell you the benefits of fasting that I have experienced. Before, I used to have many digestion problems like constipation and a bloated stomach all the time, but ever since I started fasting, these problems are gone, and my body is light.

My weight is also appropriate for my age. Ekadashi, besides physical benefits, has many mental benefits. You will feel relaxed and your mind will be calm. Moreover, it has many spiritual benefits. Fasting on Ekadashi every 15 days gives you the power to grow spiritually very fast, so I strongly recommend everyone to fast on Ekadashi day as it is an ancient tradition of great spiritual importance, especially for the Brahmacharya lifestyle.

The third rule is meditation. Many seekers have doubts and issues about meditation. The common complaint is the wandering mind when they try to meditate. People complain that their minds think about worldly matters, wandering in the market, office, cinema hall, etc.

If you are not able to meditate properly as you wish, then I have a solid suggestion that I follow in my daily life. My method of entering into complete silence is doing Bhastrikā Prāṇāyāma before meditation. Bhastrikā is done in three types of motions: Fast, medium, and slow motion. I do 100 rounds of fast motion Bhastrikā and then 100 medium and slow motion, in total 200 rounds. You can start meditation right after Bhastrika Prānāyāma. One important thing, there is a big difference between Bhastrika and Kapalbhati Prānāyāma. In Kapalbhati, there is forceful exhalation using more abdominal force, but in Bhastrika, the lungs are more active along with deep inhalation and exhalation.

Before you meditate, try this and see its amazing effects. Your mind will become quiet and peaceful in no time. This is the state of meditation without thoughts. Stay in this state for 1-2 minutes, sitting silently in "Dhyāna Mudra". This is how meditation is done.

One minute of this meditation is equal to one hour of normal meditation. Your meditation will be effortless and natural, and your mind will be calm and stable. After 2 minutes, if your mind starts to wander again, do Nadīshodhan Prānāyāma right away.

We have already taught you how to do Nadīshodhan Prānāyāma before. Do it at least 7 times. Then you will see that your breath is balanced in both nostrils. This will make your mind still and calm. All your thoughts will vanish without any effort. You will not have any thought, any distraction, any fear, any anxiety, any regret, or any attachment in this serene state. This is the higher state of meditation. You can start with 5 minutes of meditation and gradually increase the duration as you wish. Meditation is not something you do, but something that happens without effort as it is a state without thoughts. This will help you a lot to follow the Brahmacharya lifestyle and to grow spiritually faster. You can also do Nadīshodhan at night, but make sure you have a 2-hour gap after your last meal. This will help you sleep well and wake up early. This will also prevent you from having bad dreams at night. There is a lot of negative energy in the atmosphere.

I suggest that all those who want to succeed in Brahmacharya and grow spiritually should recite Hanuman Chalisa twice a day, or at least once. You should also chant one Mālā(108 times) the powerful mantra *"Om Aryamaye Namah"*, as this is a healing mantra recommended by some Spiritual Gurus especially to protect us from losing Brahmacharya and to increase the power of Brahmacharya energy. Another Mālā (108 times) is suggested in the evening and before going to bed you should chant it 21 times. This will save you from sexual dreams and nightfall. This is a practical mantra therapy as millions of Youths have experienced its unbelievable benefits and shared their testimonies on our social platforms.

According to the belief of Sanātana Dharma, chanting this mantra is a way to receive the blessings of *Aryamā Deity*, who is the leader of the ancestral beings (Pitra Loka). Aryamā Deity has the power to change our thoughts and lifestyle very quickly if we chant the above mantra with full faith and honesty. Aryamā Deity is also a form of Sun God and Lord Shri Krishna, as Lord Shri Krishna has said in Bhagwat Gīta that I am Aryamā among all the ancestors.

Finally, I will share another tip and a magical story from my life. I have noticed that 90% of Young People still need a spiritual guide or Guru. If you think you don't need a Guru, it is like sailing in a boat in the vast ocean without a navigator or a direction controller. If you have a spiritual Guru, you should practice the Guru-mantra the most.

But even if you don't, don't worry. Choose any God that you love, be it Hanuman, Lord Rama, Lord Krishna, Goddess Durga, Lord Shiva or Lord Ganesha. Pick a beautiful name for your chosen God and recite it as a mantra for at least 20-30 minutes every day.

You should chant in such a way that whenever you face the worst situation of life and you urgently need inner courage, power, and support, this Guru mantra will help you miraculously. Even when you see such a situation or disaster coming or happening, you should remember the Lord's name in less than a second. Make this your habit. This is what I experienced. Please do this for one month continuously; when such a situation or fear arises, you will remember your God's name in less than a second. This should be the strict routine of your daily prayer. You have to develop this habit gradually.

I will tell you one of my stories that happened in the year 2010. I was going to another village and riding a scooter about 45-50 km away from my hometown. There was a bridge that I had to cross on the way. On the way back, I was under the bridge on a rough road, and a four-wheeler was coming from the opposite direction. This vehicle was on my right side, and a deep valley was 40-50 feet on my left. I did not notice this deep valley when I was going, but I got scared when I saw it when I was coming back. That vehicle came fast on my right and passed, touching my right side. In that situation, my mind went blank. I did not know whether to press the brake or clutch or where to turn the handle. I got nervous. My mind was numb. There was only the name of my God on my lips. That name was the only thing I remembered, nothing else, and I fell with the scooter into the valley. I had fallen down to around 10 feet, and the scooter had fallen down to 50 feet.

You can understand. I got a minor injury in my leg. I got up with the same energy I had fallen, and I asked a passer-by for help. With the help of the passer-by, I pulled out the scooter with the same energy. The scooter was badly damaged, but I came back almost 12 km on the same scooter. I got it fixed in a garage, but it was so badly damaged that it could not be fixed completely. Then I came back to my village. I want to tell you that I did not feel any pain since I had fallen and came back home, but I can clearly remember that there was some special energy in me. I feel it because of the power of the mantra, the power of "remembrance". So many such incidents have happened in my life. The place of this accident was so dangerous that hardly anyone survived. The person who helped me said, "You don't know since you are new, but there were many accidents in this place which were usually very deadly." Everything I have written in this chapter is true and my personal experience. You must understand its importance to get a better mindset for Brahmacharya.

CHAPTER XXX

The Role of Brahmacharya in Monastic and Yogic Traditions

In this chapter, I want to explore the lives of extraordinary folk who, through the sacred vow of Brahmacharya, attained remarkable heights in their endeavors. From revered yogis to ascetic thinkers, we uncover the tales of those who embraced this commitment, achieving unparalleled success in their chosen paths. Through potent lines/verses from age-old scriptures, the chapter weaves a tapestry illustrating the transformative power of Brahmacharya on the lives of these spiritual luminaries.

"Brahmacharya tapasādeva mrityu mupāghnata"—"The Vedas state that by Brahmacharya and austerity, the Devas have overcome death."[157] How did Hanuman become a Mahāvir? With this weapon of Brahmacharya, he gained unbeatable strength and courage. The great Bhishma, the grandfather of Pāndavas and Kauravas, defeated death by Brahmacharya. Only Lakshmana, the ideal Brahmachārī, overcame the man of immense power, the ruler of three worlds, Meghanāda, son of Rāvana. It was by the power of Brahmacharya that Lakshmana could conquer the invincible Meghanāda. There is nothing in the three worlds that a Brahmachārī cannot achieve. The Rishis of old fully appreciated the value of Brahmacharya, they have written beautiful verses about the glory of Brahmacharya.

The Srutis declare: *"Nayam Ātmā balaheenena labhya—*this ātman is not attainable by a weak man." Lord Shri Krishna in Bhagwat Gīta says *"Trividham narakasyedam dvāram nāsanāmātmanah; kāmah krodhastathā lobhastasmad etat trayam tyajet—O Arjuna!* Triple is the gate of the hell, destructive of the Self; lust, wrath, and greed: therefore let man renounce these three"[158]. *"Jāhi satrum mahabaho kāmarupam durasadam—*Kill this powerful enemy, passion, by observing Brahmacharya".[159]

Just as the oil in a wick burns with bright light, the Vīrya or semen rises up by the practice of Yoga Sadhana and is transformed into Tejas or Ojas. The Brahmachārī glows with Brahmic Aurā on his face. Brahmacharya is the bright light that shines in the house of the human body. It is the fully-flowered flower of life around which the bees of strength, patience, knowledge, and purity and Dhriti wander about buzzing here and there. In other words, he who observes Brahmacharya will be blessed with the above qualities. Scriptures declare emphatically: *"Āyustejo balam veeryam prajnā shrischa yasastathā punyam cha satpriyatam cha vardhate brahmacharyayā"*—By the practice of Brahmacharya, longevity, glory, strength, vigour, knowledge, wealth, undying fame, virtues and devotion to Truth increase."

Brahmacharya is the foundation for the attainment of Kāyā Siddhi. Complete celibacy must be observed. This is of utmost importance. Through the practice of Yoga, the semen becomes transmuted into Ojas-Shakti. The Yogi will have a perfect body. There will be charm and grace in his movements. He can live as long as he likes (Icchā Mrityu). That is why Lord Krishna says to Arjuna:

"Tasmāt yogī bhavārjuna—therefore, become a Yogī, O Arjuna."

Chaste women can be called Brahmacharinis. Through the force of Brahmacharya, many women of old have done miraculous deeds and shown the world the power of chastity. Nalayanī, by the power of chastity, has stopped the sun's rising to save her husband's life. Anasuyā turned the Trimurtis— Brahmā, Vishnu, and Mahesvara into babies when they wanted Nirvana Bhiksha. Only through the power of chastity could she turn the Great Deities into babies. Savitri has brought back the life of Satyavān, her husband, from the noose of Yama by her chastity. Such is the glory of womanhood. Such is the power of chastity or Brahmacharya.

Women who lead a householder's life with chastity can also become an Anasuyā, Nalayanī, or Savitrī. Real culture is the establishment of perfect physical and mental Brahmacharya. Real culture is the realization of the identity of the individual soul with the Supreme Soul through direct experience. For a passionate worldly- minded man, the terms: 'Self-realization,' 'God, Self-Vairāgya, renunciation, death, burial ground' are very revolting and terrifying because he is attached to objects. The terms singing, dancing, and talk of ladies are very pleasing. The attraction to objects will gradually vanish if one begins to think seriously about the unreal nature of the world.

To achieve the aim of life by living purely, one must realize the grave harms of an impure life and keep his mind occupied with Divine thoughts, focus, meditation, learning, and helping others. Vedic Hindus were unbeatable because of Brahmacharya rules; they ruled the Earth 3000 years ago.

I want you to imagine your future if you follow continence for a long time. Here are some of the most valuable achievements of great men who propagated Brahmacharya in modern times.

Swamī Vivekānanda:

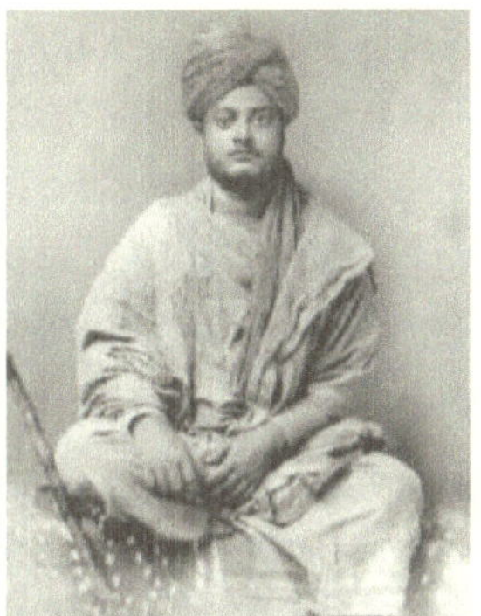

Swāmi has a special impact on the lives of people all over the world. People trust him blindly, and his words still guide them to live a peaceful life. His amazing memory power and undisturbed focus have influenced millions of lives. He has always advised youth to be celibate for at least 12 years to discover their real potential. In his short life, he has set an example for youth. This is all possible just because of celibacy. You will find some of his powerful quotes in the later chapter.

Swāmi Dayānand Saraswati:

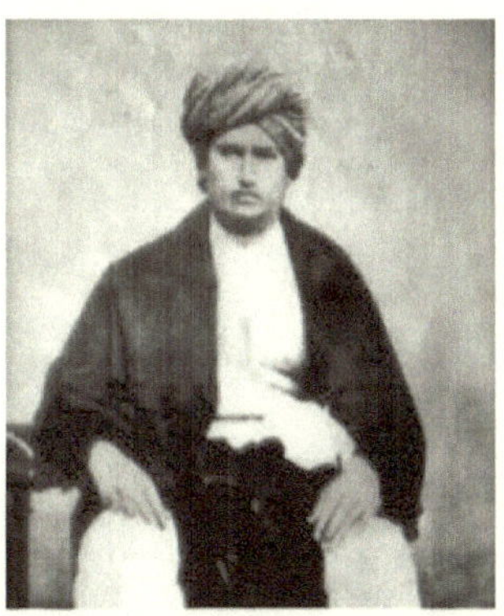

He was the first to give the call for Swaraj as "India for Indians" in 1876, a call later taken up by Lokmanya Tilak. Rejecting idolatry and ritualistic worship, he worked towards reviving Vedic ideologies. He emphasized the importance of education for all children and preached respect and equal rights for women. He founded the Ārya Samāj on April 7, 1875.

Through this reform movement, he stressed One God and rejected idol worship. He also opposed the extolled position of priests in Hinduism. Swami Dayānand Saraswati promoted the Arya Samāj movement by going to many states. People were getting impressed by him. A huge crowd used to gather in his meetings. People came from different provinces on foot, in horse or bullock carts, to listen to Swāmiji. Swāmiji's lecture was going on in one such gathering. He was giving his lecture on the topic of celibacy and was explaining its importance to the people. He was telling the people that a person who practices celibacy increases physical and intellectual strength.

The people in the meeting were listening very attentively to the words of Swāmi Dayānand Saraswati. When the meeting ended, everyone got up and started leaving. As soon as Swamiji got down from the stage and started moving forward, a person stopped him. He had brought his bullock cart. He came in front of Swamiji and started saying, 'Swami ji! You give big lectures on celibacy. Your words also impress. You are celibate, and I am a person living a family life. In this case, there is no comparison between us. Still, I do not see any difference between you and me.

Swami ji only smiled after listening to the words of the person with the bullock cart. After waiting for an answer from them, the person went ahead. Coming out, he sat on his bullock cart and started driving it. But what's this? The car was not moving from the toss. Both the bulls were pushing hard, but the cart was not moving forward. That person got upset. He could not understand anything. When he looked back, his surprise knew no bounds. He saw Swami ji holding the wheel of the bullock cart. He had realized his mistake and the power of celibacy. He got down from the bullock cart and fell at the feet of Swami ji.

Swami Rama Tirtha:

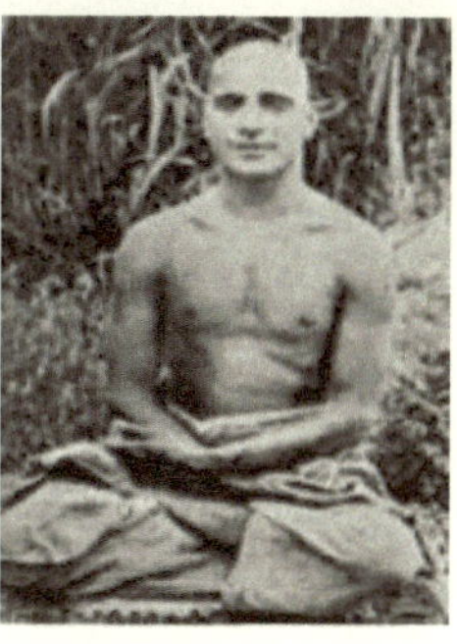

He was among the first teachers of Hinduism to lecture in the United States, traveling there in 1902, preceded by Swami Vivekananda in 1893 and followed by Paramahansa Yogānanda in 1920. During his American tours, Swami Rāma Tirtha often spoke on the concept of 'Practical Vedānta' and the education of Indian youth. He suggested bringing young Indians to American universities and helped establish scholarships for Indian students. His views on Brahmacharya were very practical; he always preferred to teach young minds the power of Yoga and knowledge of Brahmacharya.

His idea was to shape young clay, not to force hard ones. His achievements are all the grace of Brahmacharya. In the time of British rule, going to the United States and making them agree to provide scholarships to Indian students was not an easy task. This power of agreement is only possible by Brahmacharya.

Swāmi Sivānanda:

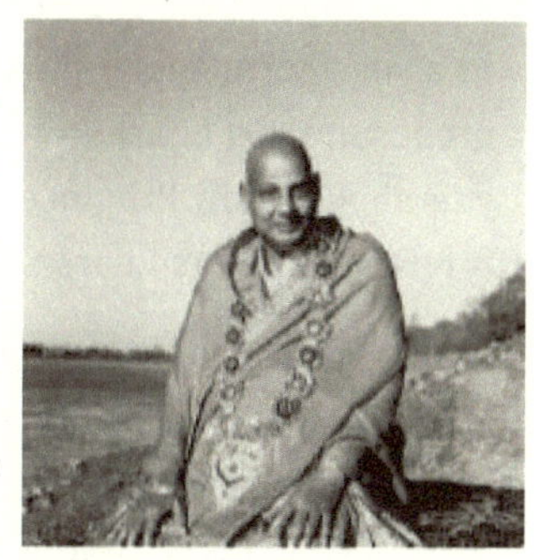

He authored 296 books on topics such as metaphysics, Yoga, Vedanta, religion, western philosophy, psychology, eschatology, fine arts, ethics, education, health, sayings, poems, epistles, autobiography, biography, stories, dramas, messages, lectures, dialogues, essays, and anthology. His books focused on the practical application of Yoga philosophy over theoretical knowledge. This task is not the task of an ordinary person. All senses must be in harmony to make such things possible. Brahmacharya is the only way to do so. I hope. It makes you feel the power of persistence in the study.

Paramhansa Yogānanda:

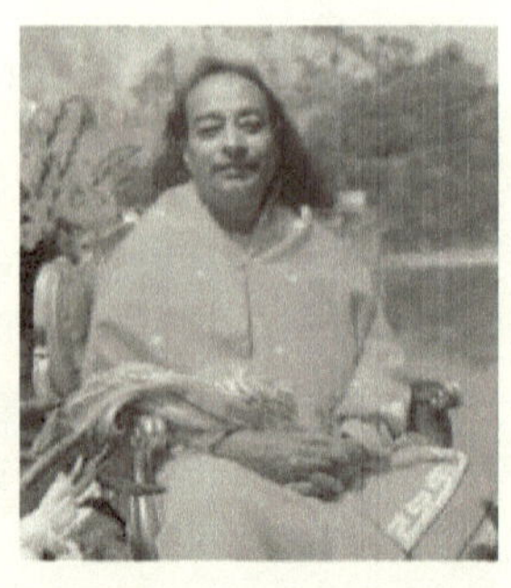

Author of the best- selling spiritual classic Autobiography of a Yogi, this beloved world teacher has introduced millions of readers to the perennial wisdom of the East. He is now widely recognized as the Father of Yoga in the West. He founded the Yogodā Satsanga Society of India in 1917 and the Self-Realization Fellowship in 1920, which continue to carry on his spiritual legacy worldwide under the leadership of Sri Sri Swāmi Chidānanda Giri, who succeeded Sri Sri Mrinalinī Mātā as the fifth president. Paramahansa Yogānanda has profoundly impacted the lives of millions with his comprehensive teachings on the science of Kriyā Yoga meditation, the underlying unity of all true religions, the art of balanced health and well-being in body, mind, and soul. All his work was so amazing that he has huge respect everywhere. Respect automatically increases with the time you have spent in Brahmacharya.

Swāmi Lilāshah Ji:

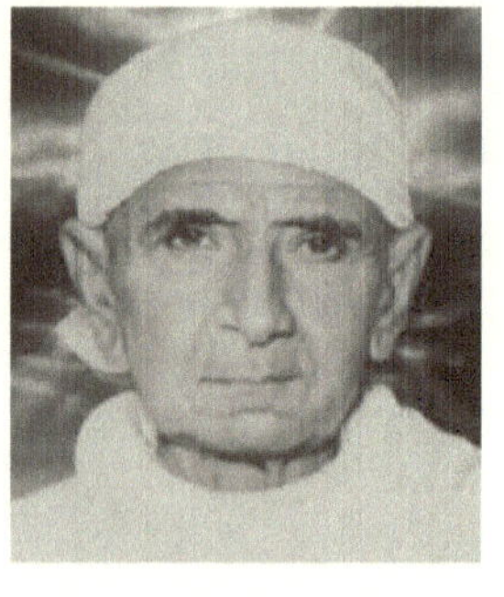

Sant Lilāshāh (Swāmi Lilāshāh) was multi-faceted. He was a yoga guru, Ayurveda physician, Vedic scholar, and a great saint. Sri Lilāshāh was born in a small village in Hyderabad, Sindh Province Pakistan In the year 1880. His birth name was Lilārām.

At a young age, his parents died, so he was brought up by his relatives. Due to his spiritual thirst, he remained a bachelor, became a Saint, and propagated the "RĀMA BHAKTI" among the people. He dedicated his life to the upliftment of the poor, oppressed and illiterate people. He was well-versed in many languages, and an expert in Vedas, Shāstras, and Hindu Purānas. He became the disciple of Sant Shri Keshavarām, and afterward, he was named Lilashāh by Muslims as he performed a yogic miracle to move a Neem tree with his mere words which was a cause of dispute among Hindu & Muslims.

He traveled to North India, visited many holy temples, performed penance in the Himalayān mountain caves, and obtained great yogic powers through that.

After some time, Swāmi returned to Sindh and published spiritual magazines. He travelled throughout India, spread the bhakti spirit among the people, and educated poor children.

He founded Annadān choultries, Cow shelters, Ayurveda Hospitals, Yoga centres, Marriage halls, and Spiritual libraries throughout India. Swamiji travelled to foreign countries and healed the people through Ayurveda medicines, started Yoga centres, and taught them Yoga and meditation. He fought for the welfare of women and conducted mass marriages at his own cost. He lived a holy and simple life.

Asharam Bapu:

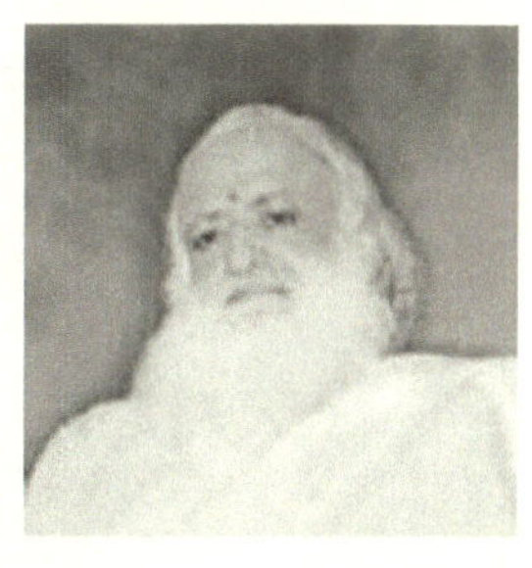

In the modern era, one of the most influential figures from the *Dādu Din Dayāl Guru* tradition is Asharam Bapu, a respected saint who has devoted the past five decades of his life to the revival and advancement of Indian Sanātan culture. A disciple of the revered Saint Swami Lilāshāh Mahārāj, Saint Ashāram Bapu has embodied the principle of Brahmacharya, placing it at the top of his teachings and actions. Through his extensive literary works, philanthropic endeavors, and enlightening discourses, Saint Asharam Bapu has undoubtedly played a key role in spreading the knowledge of Brahmacharya. His efforts have sparked a revolution in society, instilling a deep sense of celibacy among the masses. Notably, in the 1980s, he initiated a campaign called Yuvādhan Surakshā (Youth Protection Campaign), whereby a book on celibacy, initially distributed free of charge, found its way into every household, educational institution, school, and college. This noble initiative, still ongoing, has since been renamed "Divya Preraṇā Prakāsh" or "Divine Inspiration the Secret of Eternal youth" in English. To date, approximately 20 million copies of this book have been distributed both within India and overseas, transforming the lives of countless individuals who have embraced the teachings of Brahmacharya.

Furthermore, recognising the harmful impact of lust and the erosion of Brahmacharya caused by Valentine's Day, Saint Asharam Bapu initiated 'Parents' Worship Day' on February 14th. This observance aimed to prevent the degradation of youths and instill reverence and devotion among the youth towards their parents, thereby creating a new moral and cultural framework essential for the progress of any nation. The celebration of Parents' Worship Day, both within India and abroad, has facilitated the development of virtuous character traits in young individuals.

As a result, such individuals remain firm in their commitment to Brahmacharya, protecting and nurturing their inner selves. Under the inspiration of Saint Asharam Bapu, thousands of Bāla Sanskār Centers and numerous Gurukuls have been established throughout the country. These institutions provide children with comprehensive spiritual and moral education from a tender age, enabling them to effortlessly embrace celibacy until the time of marriage. Even after marriage, these individuals continue to lead lives of self-control and discipline.

Swāmi Samarth Rāmdās:

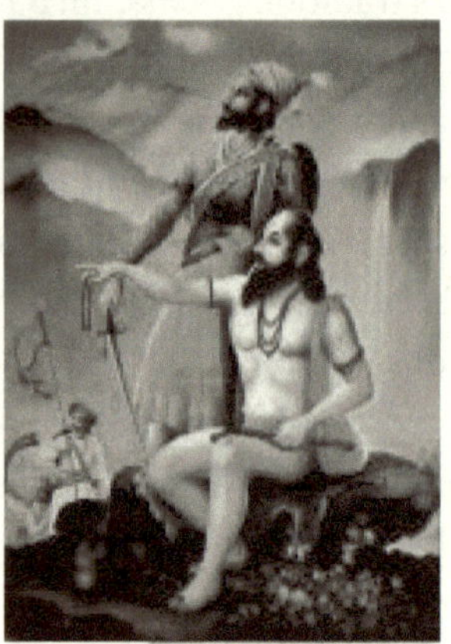

He had amazing spiritual and physical power. He has seen lord Hanuman several times because of his Brahmacharya and Sadhana. He started his Brahmacharya & Spiritual sadhana at the age of 12 years and chanted Ram nam for 12 years. He used to do 1200 Surya namaskar daily. He wrote his Ramayan and other vedic scriptures for marathi and hindi readers. After that he started visiting other states of India for 12 years on foot. At 36, he reached the Himalayas and thought to take vairagya by leaving his body. This was his satisfaction with life. He jumped from 1000 ft, but Lord Ram saved him and asked him to do holy things and spread awareness of God. There are many magical stories about him but. This is enough to understand how powerful Brahmacharya is. He was the guru of Shivāji Mahārāj and taught him the religious practices and ideas of Hindu Rāshtra.

I have done my best to inspire you by telling you the importance of Brahmacharya. But the benefits of Brahmacharya and the superhuman people who have experienced it are also endless. We express our gratitude and respect to countless such souls whose names we could not mention in this book but they followed Brahmacharya and did great works for humanity. We can only cover a few things in a small book. This book will fill you with immense enthusiasm to follow celibacy if you sincerely read and apply it. Make a habit of learning more and more about the above-mentioned great men for continuous increase in knowledge and faith about Brahmacharya.

Let's read some of the most powerful quotes on Brahmacharya in the next chapter.

CHAPTER XXXI

Inspiring Quotes And Thoughts

Swami Vivekananda: Power comes to him, who observes unbroken Brahmacharya for twelve years. Complete continence gives great intellectual and spiritual power. Controlled desire leads to the highest results. Transform sexual energy into spiritual energy. The stronger this force, the more can be done with it. Only a powerful current of water can do hydraulic mining. Simply by the observance of strict Brahmacharya (continence), all learning can be mastered quickly — one has an unfailing memory of what one hears or knows but once. Due to this want of continuity, everything is on the brink of ruin in our country. If a person can be on a continent for twelve years, he can have extraordinary memories. One must be celibate and keep his Brahmacharya even in his dream." Our motherland requires some of her children to become such pure-souled Brahmacharis and Brahmacharinis.

Shri Ramakrishna Paramahansa: To be able to realize God, one must practice absolute continence. A man practicing unbroken Brahmacharya for twelve years develops a special power. When a man succeeds in conserving his sexual energy, his intellect reflects the image of Brahman. If you want to realize God, you must be a Brahmachari. Without practicing Brahmacharya, one cannot concentrate steadily on God. The loss of reproductive elements dissipates a person's strength. They squander it all by breaking Brahmacharya. That's why they can't hold on to spiritual instruction. You have to clean yourself of the dirt of 'lust and greed.

Shri Aurobindo: By practicing Brahmacharya, they devoted all the energy that the system had and that was not needed for bodily functions to the brain. In this way, they not only enhanced mental strength, or the power of grasping, or the mind, or the subtlety and quickness of thinking, the memory and the creative intellectual force that made the triple force of memory, invention, and judgment complete and analytic, but they also greatly expanded the scope, as well as the intensity, of the mental activities that could absorb, store, and generate. The practice of Brahmacharya is the first and most essential condition of increasing the force inside and using it for such purposes as may benefit the owner or humanity.

Other Inspiring Quotes on Brahmacharya :

- Brahmacharya is abstaining from all kinds of *Maithuna* or sexual enjoyment forever, in all places and all conditions, physically, mentally, and verbally – Yājnavalkya.

- Thinking of a woman or her picture, praising a woman or her picture, sporting with a woman or her picture, glancing at a woman or her picture, secretly talking to a woman, thinking of a sinful action towards a woman actuated by sensuality, determining upon the sinful action, and bodily action resulting in the discharge of semen is the eight characteristics of copulation. Brahmacharya is quite contrary to all these eight indications- *Daksha Smriti.*

- Know that nothing can be unattained by one who remains from birth to death a perfect celibate. In one person, knowledge of the four Vedas, and in another, perfect celibacy—of these, the latter is superior to the former who is leaving in celibacy- *The Mahābhārata.*

- Brahmacharya or spotless chastity is the best of all penances; a celibate of such spotless chastity is not a human being, but a god indeed. To the celibate who conserves semen with great effort, what is there unattainable in this world? By the power of the composure of the semen, one will become just like me - *Lord Shankara.*

- Those students who find that world of God through chastity, theirs is that heavenly country; theirs, in whatever world they are, is freedom - *Chhandogya Upanishad.*

- A wise man should avoid married life as if it were a burning pit of live coals. From the contact comes sensation, from sensation thirst, from thirst clinging; by ceasing from that, the soul is delivered from all sinful existence - *Lord Buddha.*

- These sexual propensities, though they are at first like ripples, acquire the proportions of a sea on account of bad company – *Nārada Muni.*

- Sensuality destroys life, luster, strength, vitality, memory, wealth, great fame, holiness and devotion to the Supreme - *Lord Krishna.*

- Death is hastened by letting out semen from the body; life is saved and prolonged by preserving it. There is no doubt that people die prematurely by letting semen out of the body; knowing this, the Yogi should always preserve semen and lead a life of strict celibacy - *Shiva Samhitā.*

- Caution in the diet is of threefold value, but abstinence from sexual intercourse is of fourfold value. The Sannyāsi had, and has, a rule never to look at a woman *–Maharshi Atreya.*

- Let not a Brahmin see a woman naked *–Manu Rishi.*

- For there are some eunuchs, which were born from their Mother's womb; there are some eunuchs of men; and there are eunuchs, which made themselves eunuchs for the kingdom of heaven's sake. He can receive it. – *FromBible(Math. xix. 12)* "Do not say that you have a chaste mind if your eyes are unchaste because an unchaste eye betrays an unchaste heart- *St. Augustine, Jesus Christ.*

- The spiritual life starts with recognizing that as long as you keep going headlong to pursue a sense of satisfaction and pleasure, you will not move one step - *Swami Chidananda.*

- There appears to be a need for some bold man who will say outright what is best ... Opposing the mightiest lusts and following reason only - *Plato , Laws, VIII , 835.*

- Stressing physical science without corresponding cultivation of spiritual factors has lowered man's sense of moral power and responsibility - *Sockman , Morals Of Tomorrow, I , III, 68.*

- In the process of that growth, all humanity must conquer passion must gradually diminish the abuse of sex. Man as you are today half man half beast. . . Are you so satisfied with your bastard and imperfect humanity with your penalty scarcely held on a leash? - *Papini , Life Of Christ, 123*

- There is a small organ in the human body which is always hungry if one tries to satisfy it, and always satisfied if one starves it -*The Talmud, Sanhedrin, 107A; Quoted In : Talmey , Love, XXIV, 403.*

- Whatever is given to the body is taken from the spirit - *Kingsford, The Perfect Way, VM , 217.*

- When once you have escaped the violence of this secret destruction implanted in your very vitals, every other desire will pass you by un-harmed - *Seneca ,*

"To Helvia On Consolation", XIII, 3; In His Moral Essay.

- Sexual intercourse involves the destruction of our bodies, the shortening of life – *Aristotle.*

- What Brahmacharya means is a deep clarity about sexual energy - *Judith Hanson Lasater, Ph.D.*

- People often get confused about this. They always think it's the seminal discharge that's undesirable, but it's actually the firing of the nervous system during sexual stimulation. And that applies to both men and women - *Georg Feuerstein.*

- To make the most of the evolutionary advantages and possibilities it is evident that the first place youth, up to full maturity, should conserve all of life's energy for the development of body and of brain - *Adolescence, Ch.XXIV*

- At that time when mankind became accustomed and addicted to sexual acts without reproductive purpose, at that very time it put a deadlock into the course of its evolution. Not until this deadlock is removed can humanity, individually and jointly , stride on toward the attainment of the greater faculties and powers which evolution has in store for man - *The Future, Chapter.LXXXIV*

- Man's truly godlike possession lies in the possibility of spiritual development. Not in sex. On the contrary, "the absolutely spiritual man is . . . entirely disconnected from sex"- *BLAVATSKY , The Secret Doctrine, III , 438.*

- Sexual action that is not propagative cannot be considered to be in harmony with nature's purposes. Every attempt to justify unreproductive sexual action can only be the result of a wish to whitewash the addiction of humanity to sexual abuse - *Perversion, Chapter XXIX*

- Where animals are only sexual, man has become sensual by degrading the reproductive sexual urge into a desire for unreproductive sensual satisfaction. Sensuality is man-made. By overexciting the reproductive faculty for millions of years man has only himself to blame for the impelling power of the sexual impulse. And only he himself can reduce that power and bring it back within the boundaries of its legitimate domain: that of the perpetuation of the race. - *The Coiled Serpent, Chapter on Instinct*

- There are great "artists who feel most fit for work when refraining entirely from sexual intercourse"- *SENATOR - KAMINER , Health and Disease, ii, 20.*

- There are couples who . . . give up sexual relations absolutely, and are not, any less happy, but often more happy on that account" - *ROBINSON, America's Sex, Marriage and Divorce Problems, IX , 411*

- In order to remove the greatest obstacle to the improvement of the race "man must assume a more complete restraint over his reproductive functions and subordinate his inclinations to the future interests of his descendants" - *MARSHALL, Introduction to Sexual Physiology, VIII, 148.*

- The intellectual life of a whole nation must suffer if sexual activity is the rule among its young people - *POPENOE , Conservation of the Family, II , ii, 63*

- So much of the life force is then wasted on the sexual level that none can be transformed into the higher energy on which aspiration and idealism depend. Thus "continence...is connected with ideal aspirations no less than with physical vigour" **HASTINGS , Encycl. of Religion and Ethics, III , 484** and with mental clarity. Therefore the way to maintain a strong and pure idealism through life is to adhere to continence - *The Coiled Serpent, Ch. Adolescent*

- Under conditions of right thinking and right living the seminal fluid would be produced only when there is a demand for propagation - *ARMITAGE , Sex Force, III , ii , 17.*

- Every expression of the sexual impulse that does not correspond with nature's purpose of propagation must be regarded as perverse. - *KRAFFT-EBING , Psychopathia Sexualis,*

- The person who shows sex abnormalities is potentially the most dangerous casual criminal - *COOPER , Here's to Crime, XIV, 293.*

- The more continently one lives the better work one can produce, because in body and in mind "energy is gained by the establishment of continence - *Patanjali, Yoga Sutras, II, 38*

- The tradition of sex necessity is a dangerous lie, particularly as it is founded on the false assumption that cohabitation is essential to health

- *COWAN , The Science of a New Life, XXIII, 243*

- Every use of the sexual function beyond intended race- preservation constitutes a misuse, an excess. And "excess . . . brings on disease, misery, suffering, mental and physical - *The Mahatma Letters, X, 57*

- It is largely through the abuse of the sex force that "man is more diseased. . . than any animal" - *NIETZSCHE,, Genealogy of Morals, III , 13.*

- Continence would be of the greatest help in humanity's struggle against illness, because in the continent person the undiminished internal secretions *- Glands and Secretions, Chapter XXIV*

- Choose rather to be strong in soul than in body - *IAMBLICHUS , Life of Pythagoras, 186*

- Having put aside the habit and thought of sexual intercourse, his life is pure - *BECK , The Splendour of Asia, xvii, 210*

- To be carnally minded is death, but to be spiritually minded is life - *Romans, VIII, 6*

- Spiritual comforts exceed all the delights of the world and all pleasures of the flesh - *THOMA S A KEMPIS , Imitation of Christ, II , x, 1.*

- Abstinence leads to purity and purity leads to holiness - *The Talmud, Abodah Zarah, 20b; VII, 220*

- Spiritual wisdom is the fruit of indifference to sensual pleasures. - *Adhyatma Upanishad, I, 5*

- *The supreme mystery of the Vedas is not to be declared to those whose senses are not subdued - Svetasvatara Upanishad,VI , 22 ; in : Sacred Books of the East, XV , 267. See also: Maitri Upanishad, VI , 29; and Brihad-Aranyaka Upanishad, VI , iii, 12*

- Cut down the whole forest of lust! When you have cut down every tree and every shrub, then you will be free! - *BUDDHA , Dhammapada, XX, 283*

- Only he who knows that lusts have a short taste and cause pain, is wise

- *Dhammapada, XIV , 186; in : Sacred Books of the East, X (I) , 51.*

- *Freedom from lust . . . this truly is the highest happiness -Mahavagga, I , III, 3; in : Sacred Books of the East, XIII , 85*

- When the inward fires of lust are extinguished, then one has entered into Nirvana. This is the Lesson of Lessons - *BECK, The Splendour of Asia, XVIII, 226*

- He who rejoices in the objects of senses and passions is like a thirsty man drinking poison to quench his thirst - *SANKARACHARYA, Mahavakyadarpanam, 207; in : The Theosophist, XIV , 18*

- If you long ardently for liberation, put sensuous desires away - *SANKARACHARYA , The Crest Jewel of Wisdom, 84.*

- Only if "freed from passion . . . and purified in the fire of wisdom, men have entered into a realization of the Supreme - *Bhagavad Gita, IV, 10.*

- The main end and design of Pythagoras philosophy was to disengage the mind from the bonds of the body - *DACIER, Life of Pythagoras. 29*

- *Continence precedes the acquisition of every good - DEMOPHILUS, Pythagoric Sentences"; in: SALLUST, On the Gods and the World, 111.*

- *Nature produced the seed for the sake of producing children, and not for the sake of lust - GHAROXDAS . "Preface to a Treatise of Laws": in : TAYLOR , Political Fragments of Ancient Pythagoreans, 45.*

- Socrates exhorted his companions to practise self-control in the matter of sexual indulgence - *Xenophon;. Memorabilia, II . ii. 1*

- We make the nearest approach to wisdom when we . . . are not surfeited with the bodily nature but keep ourselves pure - *Plato*

- Avoid the inclinations to animalistic pleasure, for . . . such pleasure brings with it stains on the soul - *Aristotle, Secreta Secretorum, , IX ; quoted in : Bacon , Opus Majus, II , 680.*

- The self-restrained man stands firm against passion - *Aristotle, Nicomachean Ethics, VII , IX, 2.*

- The cause of disharmony and of an unhappy life is that men follow .. . the lower animal principle and let it run away with them - *Bevan , Stoics and Sceptics, III, 103*

- Sexual desire has been given to man not for the gratification of pleasure but for the continuance of the human race - *SENECA, "To Helvia on Consolation", xiii, 3; in his Moral Essays. II , 463.*

- Spirituality is conditioned by ... a temperament disciplined into chastity and renunciation - *SANTAYANA , Platonism and the Spiritual Life, xi, 38.*

- The flesh is strong only in the weakness of the spirit *-SOLOVYOP , Justification of the Good, I , ii, 47*

- Supremacy of the spirit over the flesh is necessary in order to preserve the moral dignity of man - *SOLOVYOP, Justification of the Good, I , ii, 57*

- The true good becomes more and more discernible . . . after one recognizes that sensual pleasure is only a hindrance - *SPINOZA, On the Improvement of the Understanding; in his Chief Works, II , 6.*

- To control the sexual impulse efficiently has always been and ever will be regarded as the highest test of human wisdom - *COMTE , System of Positive Polity, III , 380*

- The sexual impulse appears as a malevolent demon that strives to pervert, confuse and overthrow everything - *SCHOPENHAUER , The World as Will and Idea, IV , xliv, 339 .*

- Animals we are and animals we remain, and the path to our regeneration and happiness, if there be such a path, lies through our animal nature - *RUSSELL , (Mrs.), The Right to be Happy, VI, 241*

- By the transmutation of metals the alchemists meant the conversion of man from a lower to a higher order of existence, from a natural to a spiritual life *-HITCHCOCK , Alchemy and the Alchemists, 280*

- At least half the world's misery is in some way...connected with the sexual sphere."- *ROBINSON, Sexual Problems of Today*

- The study of Yoga is impossible in the scattered condition of thoughts, desires and feelings amidst which an ordinary person lives - *OUSPENSKY, A New Model of the Universe, VI, 248.*

- Yogis know that sex energy must be conserved and used for the development of body and mind instead of being dissipated - *RAMACHARAKA , The Hindu Science of Breath, IX, 38*

- The sooner the animal sexual affinities are given up . . . the sooner will come the manifestation of the higher occult powers - *BLAVATSKY , "The Future Occultist" ; in : The Theosophist, V, 264*

- It is not death that makes reproduction necessary, but reproduction has death as its inevitable consequence -*GOETTE, Ueber den Ursprung des Todes, iii, 52*

- *He who will conquer sex will conquer death -MEREJKOWSKI , The Secret of the West, II , viii, 322*

- Immortality is the secret of transmutation - *KINGSFORB , Clothed with the Sun, I , xx, 90*

- To the man or woman who resolutely pursues the path of purity... will come unfailingly the consciousness of immortality -*PRYSE , The Apocalypse Unsealed, 82.*

- All the great teachers of the world are agreed in protesting against the dominion of appetite in the life of man - *BLACK , Culture and Restraint, vi, 147.*

- Sexual purification is a requisite for the harmoniously balanced physical, moral, mental and spiritual development of the race - *The Coiled Serpent, Ch. Epilogue.*

CHAPTER XXXII

Final Thoughts

As you reach the final pages of this transformative guide, remember that you hold within your hands not just a book, but a beacon—a guiding light that illuminates the path toward a superhuman existence.

Brahmacharya, once practised by ancient seekers of spiritual progress, now beckons to us anew. In a world fraught with challenges—sexual crises, diseases, moral decay—we stand at a crossroads. The choice is ours: to falter or to rise.

Within these sacred words lie solutions—the keys to reclaiming our inherent strength. Imagine a life where the body thrives, the mind soars, and the spirit dances. Picture a society unshackled from the burdens of lust, teenage pregnancy, and degradation. Envision a future where humanity evolves not merely to survive, but to transcend—to become suprahuman.

Scientists, Rishis, saints, and spiritual Gurus have left footprints on this path. Their remarkable qualities echo through time, urging us onward. As you close this book, let their legacy infuse your every step.

And beyond these pages, explore the digital realm. Visit the YouTube Channel **ManthanHub**, where wisdom flows in over 600 videos. There, the essence of Brahmacharya awaits—a sole guide for your life's journey. Also, you can visit this website (https://selfdefinition.org/celibacy) to download valuable books on the topic.

May your efforts bear fruit, and may you emerge not just as a survivor, but as a conqueror—a living testament to the evolution of mankind.

With unwavering resolve,
Radheshyam More

Remember, dear reader that the journey continues beyond these words. May you walk it with purpose, courage, and the fire of transformation.

Important Details :

Website : www.manthanhub.com , www.manthanhub.in

YouTube Channel (Hindi): https://www.youtube.com/@manthanhub

YouTube Channel (English): https://www.youtube.com/@thesuper humanlifestyle

Contact/ Emails: brainrewire@manthanhub.com , manthanhubservices@gmail. com

Instagram : https://www.instagram.com/manthanhub/

ManthanHub offers **brain rewiring audio sessions** that empower individuals to overcome sexual addictions, porn addiction, and mental health challenges. Available in both Hindi and English, this transformative program guides participants toward complete mental recovery and a superhuman lifestyle. For more information, visit the ManthanHub website or connect with the author directly.

CHAPTER XXXIII

References

1. Unprotected by Dr Miriam Grossman

2. The Role of Celibacy in Spiritual Life by Swami Chidanandda

3. Science Discovers the Physiological Value of Continence, By RW Bernard, Page 1 Source link - https://selfdefinition.org/celibacy/bernard/contents.htm

4. Ibid, Page 2

5. Ibid, Page 2

6. Ibid, Page 2

7. Ibid, Page 3

8. Ibid, Page 5

9. Ibid, Page 5

10. Practice of Brahmacharya By Swami Shivananda, Page 21

11. Sushruta Samhita, Chapter 14, Verse 10 and Atrideva, Atrideva; Ghanekar, Bhaskar Govindji; Vaidya, Lalchandraji (2007), Motilal Banarsidass Publishers Pvt. Limited. P 50

12. Textbook of Medical Physiology, 11th Edition, Guyton, Page 997

13. Semen Retention Miracle By Joseph Peterson, Page 22

14. Conservation Therapy By Mark Jaqua, Page 3

15. Ibid

16. Ibid

17. Ibid

18. Conservation Therapy By Mark Jaqua, Page 4

19. Science Discovers the Physiological Value of Continence, By RW Bernard, Page 5

20. Ibid, Page 6

21. Ibid, Page 6 & 7

22. Ibid, Page 9

23. Ibid, Page 10

24. Ibid

25. Ibid, Page 11

26. Ibid

27. Ibid, Page 12

28. Ibid, Page 14

29. Ibid, Page 15

30. Ibid

31. Ibid, Page 16

32. Ibid, Page 17

33. Ibid, Page 41

34. Ibid, Page 40

35. Ibid, Page 43

36. Ibid, Page 36

37. Ibid

38. Ibid

39. Ibid, Page 37

40. Ibid, Page 22

41. Ibid, Page 37

42. Ibid

43. Ibid, Page 38

44. Ibid, Page 32

45. Ibid, Page 30

46. Ibid, Page 27

47. Ibid, Page 28

48. Ibid, Page 21

49. https://www.forbes.com/health/mind/mental-health-statistics/

50. Sexually Active Teenagers Are More Likely To Be Depressed and To Attempt Suicide. A Report of the Heritage Center for Data Analysis By Robert E. Rector, Kirk A. Johnson, Lauren R. Noyes Source - https://www.researchgate.net/publication/234738096

51. An Unacknowledged Harm of Masturbation By Michael Shelton MS, LPC https://www.psychologytoday.com/intl/blog/sex-life-the-american-male/201403/unacknowledged-harm-masturbation

52. Your Brain and Masturbation By Reclaim Team #R015 - https://www.reclaimsexualhealth.com/pdfs-to-share

53. H.P. Blavatsky, The Secret Doctrine, Pasadena, CA: Theosophical University Press (TUP), 1977 (1888), 2:411.

54. 'Sexually transmitted infections (STIs)', https://www.who.int/news-room/fact-sheets/detail/sexually-transmitted-infections-(stis) And Infection risks associated with oral sex', 1 March 2016, http://www.netdoctor.co.uk/conditions/sexual-health/a12020/infection-risks-associated-with-oral-sex

55. webmd.com/sexual-conditions/guide/sexual-health-stds;webmd.com/genital-herpes/guide/what-is-it; webmd.com/sexual-conditions/guide/genital-warts.

56. cdc.gov/msmhealth/std.htm; cdc.gov/std/life-stages-populations/stdfact-msm.htm.

57. Public Health England, Promoting the health and wellbeing of gay, bisexual and other men who have sex with men, 2014, p. 7, gov.uk.

58. 'The birth control pill: a history', June 2015, plannedparenthood.org; 'Are there side effects of birth control pills?', webmd.com.

59. Ashley Welch, 'Report finds nearly half of all abortions worldwide are unsafe', 27 Sep 2017, cbsnews.com.

60. D.A. Grimes et al., 'Unsafe abortion: the preventable pandemic', Sexual and Reproductive Health 4, World Health Organization, Oct 2006, who.int.

61. 'Possible physical side effects after abortion', americanpregnancy.org; 'Abortion emotional side effects', americanpregnancy.org.

62. 'Pornography statistics', familysafemedia.com.

63. Yourbrainonporn.com.

64. nofap.com; reddit.com/r/NoFap.

65. Havelock Ellis, Psychology of Sex, New York: Mentor, 1963, pp. 28-30. 'The dark side of the big "O"', 2011, sexualhealthsite.info; Marnia Robinson and Gary Wilson, 'Men: Does frequent ejaculation cause a hangover?', reuniting. info; Marnia Robinson and Gary Wilson, 'Women: Does orgasm give you a hangover?', reuniting.info; Marnia Robinson, Peace Between the Sheets: Healing with sexual relationships, Berkeley, CA: Frog, 2004; Walter Last, 'Healing with sexual energy: sex for health, relationships and spirituality', health-science-spirit.com.

66. Lauren Slater, 'True love', National Geographic, Feb 2006, nationalgeographic.com.

67. Gabrielle Brown, The New Celibacy: A journey to love, intimacy, and good health in a new age, New York: McGraw-Hill, 2nd ed., 1989, pp. 8-9 (see section 9, 'Chastity links').

68. Liz Hodgkinson, Sex is Not Compulsory, London: Sphere Books, 1988, PP. 8-9. http://www.lizhodgkinson.com/lifesexx.htm

69. Aarathi Prasad, Like a Virgin: How science is redesigning the rules of sex, Oxford: Oneworld, 2012, p. 33; Raymond W. Bernard, Science Discovers the Physiological Value of Continence, Mokelumne Hill, CA: Health Research, 1957 (see 'Chastity links').

70. Donald E. Tyler, The Other Guy's Sperm: The cause of cancers and other diseases, Ontario, OR: Discovery Books, 1994 (see 'Chastity links').

71. 'Prostatitis', patient.info/doctor/prostatitis.

72. Edwin Flatto, Warning: Sex may be hazardous to your health, New York: Arco, 2nd ed., 1977, pp. 29-40 (see 'Chastity links'); Edwin Flatto, Super Potency at Any Age, New York: Thorsons, 1993, pp. 37-44.

73. R.B. Hayes et al., 'Sexual behaviour, STDs and risks for prostate cancer', British Journal of Cancer, v. 82, 2000, pp. 718-25, ncbi.nlm.nih.gov; K.A. Rosenblatt et al., 'Sexual factors and the risk of prostate cancer', American Journal of Epidemiology, v. 153, 2001, pp. 1152-8, ncbi.nlm.nih.gov; L.K. Dennis and D.V. Dawson, 'Meta-analysis of measures of sexual activity and prostate cancer', Epidemiology, v. 13, 2002, pp. 72-9, ncbi.nlm.nih.gov.

74. G.G. Giles et al., 'Sexual factors and prostate cancer', BJU International, v. 92, 2003, pp. 211-6, blackwell-synergy.com; Comment on Giles et al. by S. Brody, blackwell-synergy.com; Comment on Giles et al. by R.T.D. Oliver, blackwell-synergy.com; Douglas Fox, 'Masturbating may protect against prostate cancer', 16 July 2003, newscientist.com.

75. Ibid

76. Raymond Bernard, The Physiological Enigma of Woman: The mystery of menstruation, Health Research, n.d.; Hilton Hotema, Secret of Regeneration, Health Research, 1963, ch. 179-185, 188- 189.

77. Sex is Not Compulsory, pp. 167-75; Raymond W. Bernard, Nutritional Sex Control & Rejuvenation, Health Research, n.d.; Swami Sivananda, Practice of Brahmacharya, 1997, P 18, sivanandadlshq.org.

78. Elizabeth Abbott, A History of Celibacy, New York: Scribner, 2000, P 85.

79. Warning: Sex may be hazardous to your health, By Dr Edwin Flatto, PP 133-4.

80. Ibid., P 17; Secret of Regeneration, Ch. 193.

81. Emily Walker-Monash, 'Sperm production is costly, crickets show', 31 January 2012, futurity.org.

82. A.T. Barker (comp.), The Mahatma Letters to A.P. Sinnett, TUP, 2nd ed., 1975, pp. 122, 274 / Wheaton, IL: Theosophical Publishing House (TPH), chron. ed., 1993, pp. 161, 137; The Secret Doctrine, 2:295-6; H.P. Blavatsky Collected Writings, TPH, 1950-91, 12:702.

83. G. de Purucker, The Esoteric Tradition, TUP, 3rd ed., 2013, pp. 495-6; H.S. Olcott, Old Diary Leaves, TPH, 1974, 2:218.

84.   The Secret Doctrine by Helena Blavatsky, 2:302.

85.   G. de Purucker, Man in Evolution, TUP, 2nd ed., 1977, P.202-4.

86.   Practice of Brahmacharya by Swami Sivananda, page 19

87.   Practice of Brahmacharya by Swami Sivananda, Page 78

88.   The Gospel of Sri Ramakrishna by Mahendranath Gupta, P. 436

89.   Raymond Bernard, Nutritional Sex Control & Rejuvenation, Mokelumne Hill, CA: Health Research, n.d. (see 'Chastity links'). Link https://davidpratt.info/sex.htm#s9

90.   Maulana Abdullah Ismail, Madrasah Arabia Islamia, Azaadville South Africa. Source: archive.org/details/MasturbationByShaykhAbdullahIsmail

91.   Office of Juvenile Justice and Delinquency Prevention, Juvenile Justice Bulletin, December 2009

92.   Torkom Saraydarian (1917–1997) about Sex, Family and the Woman in Society, https://en.wikipedia.org/wiki/Torkom_Saraydarian

93.   Warning: Sex may be hazardous to your health! by Dr Edwin Flatto; New York: Arco, 2nd ed., 1977. Link: https://davidpratt.info/flatto.htm#10

94.   Ibid

95.   Ibid

96.   Ibid

97.   The American Sex Revolution by Pitirim Sorokin, Page 56

98.   Ibid, Page 59

99.   Ibid, Page 60

100.   Ibid, Page 61

101.   Ibid

102.   Ibid

103.   Ibid

104.   Modern Biological Theory & Experiment on Celibacy, Jatin Shankar

105.   Ibid

106.   Sane Sex Order By Pitrim Sorokin

107.   The American Sex Revolution, Pitirim A. Sorokin, PP 106-130

108.   Unicef (2001) A league table of teenage births in rich nations, Innocenti Report Card No 3, Florence: Innocenti Research Centre.

109.   Arney, W.R. and Bergen, B.J. (1984) 'Power and visibility –The Invention of Teenage Pregnancy, Social Science & Medicine, vol 18, no 1, pp 11-9

110.   Furstenberg, F.F., Jr (1991) 'As the pendulum swings: teenage childbearing and social concern', Family Relations, vol 40, no 2, pp 127–38.

111.   Wong, J. (1997) 'The "making" of teenage pregnancy', International Studies in the Philosophy of Science, vol 11, no 3, pp 273–88.

112.   Selman, P. (1998/2001) 'Teenage pregnancy, poverty and the welfare debate in Europe and the United States, Paper presented at the seminar Poverty, fertility and family planning, Mexico City, Mexico, 2–4 June 1998.

113.   Macleod, C. (2003) 'Teenage pregnancy and the construction of adolescence: scientific literature in South Africa', Childhood, vol 10, no 4, pp 419–37.

114.   Selman, P. (1998/2001) 'Teenage pregnancy, poverty and the welfare debate in Europe and the United States, Paper presented at the seminar Poverty, fertility and family planning, Mexico City, Mexico, 2–4 June 1998.

115.   SEU (Social Exclusion Unit) (1999) Teenage pregnancy, London: The Stationery Office.

116.   Singh, S. and Darroch, J.E. (2000) 'Adolescent pregnancy and childbearing: levels and trends in developed countries, Family Planning Perspectives, vol 31, no 1, pp 14–23.

117.   Chandola, T., Coleman, D.A. and Hiorns, R.W. (2001) Heterogeneous fertility patterns in the English-speaking world. Results from Australia, Canada, New Zealand and the United States, presentation, EAPS Population Conference, Helsinki, 7–9 June.

118.   SEU (Social Exclusion Unit) (1999) Teenage pregnancy, London: The Stationery Office.

119.   Whitehead, E. (2001) 'Teenage pregnancy: on the road to social death', International Journal of Nursing Studies, vol 38, no 4, pp 437–46.

120.   ONS (2007) Population trends 130 – births in England and Wales 2006, London: The Stationery Office.

121.   Cunnington, A.J. (2001) 'What's so bad about teenage pregnancy?', The Journal of Family Planning & Reproductive Health Care, vol 27, no 1, pp 36–41 And Breheny, M. and Stephens, C. (2007b) 'Irreconcilable differences: Health professionals' constructions of adolescence and motherhood', Social Science & Medicine, vol 64, no 1, pp 112–24.

122.   Knudsen, L.B. and Valle, A.-K. (2006) 'Teenage reproductive behaviour in Denmark and Norway: lessons from the Nordic welfare state', in A. Daguerre and C. Nativel (eds) When children become parents: The welfare state responses to teenage pregnancy, Bristol: The Policy Press, pp 161–81.

123.   Jones, E.F., Darroch Forrest, J., Goldman, N., Henshaw, S., Lincoln, R., Rosoff, J.I., Westoff, C.F. and Wulf, D. (1986) Teenage pregnancy in industrialized countries, Alan Guttmacher Institute, New Haven, CT: Yale University Press.

124.   Bennett, S.E. and Assefi, N.P. (2005) 'School-based teenage pregnancy prevention programs: a systematic review of randomized controlled trials', Journal of Adolescent Health, vol 36, no 1, pp 72–81.

125.   DCLG (Department for Communities and Local Government) (2007) Common themes: Local Strategic Partnerships and teenage pregnancy, London: DCLG. Page 6

126.   BBC News Online (2006) 'Blair to tackle "menace" children', BBC News Online, 31 August. Available online at: http://news.bbc.co.uk/1/hi/uk_politics/5301824.stm [accessed 29 October 2008].

127.   The Sex Industrial Complex, Judith A. Reisman, Ph.D. The Institute for Media Education Author, Kinsey, Crimes & Consequences (2003), Draft Report- The Indiana State Legislature, Ways and Means Committee, February 2005. (Read Executive Summary)

128.   Ibid

129. Ibid

130. Ibid

131.   Ibid

132. Ibid

133. Ibid

134.   The embattled Catholic American Thinker. Welcome to America's Protected Billion-Dollar Masturbation Industry. https://catholicamericanthinker.commasturbation-industry.html)

135. American Sex Revolution by Pitirim Sorokin, page 19

136. The Psychological Society by Martin L . Gross, page 6

137. American Sex Revolution by Pitirim Sorokin

138. Source Link - http://www.nytimes.com/2010/05/27/health/policy/27 contraceptive.html?_r=0

139. Shrimad Bhagavad gita 7.11

140. Shrimad Bhagavatam, 11.5.13

141. Innocenti Report Card 3, July 2001 Issued by UNICEF

142. American Sex Revolution by Pitirim Sorokin

143. The Coil Serpent by C. J. VanVliet (Chapter 23 on Eugenics)

144. The Autobiography of a Yogi, Paramahansa Yogananda

145. American Sex Revolution by Pitirim Sorokin, P 124

146. Ibid, Page 94

147. The Coil Serpent by C. J. VanVliet (Chapter 23 on Eugenics) And Brahmacharya Vivek by Babu Kailasnath Bhargav, Page-423

148. Brahma-Randhra: The Evolving Center in the Brain, Michael Bradford   https://www.icrcanada.org/research/kundalinievolution/brahmarandhra

149. Brahma-Randhra: The Evolving Center in the Brain, Michael Bradford https://www.icrcanada.org/research/kundalinievolution/brahmarandhra

150. The role of Celibacy in Spiritual life by Swami Chidananda.

151. Bhagwan - The God that failed" by Hugh Milne, Chapter - Life After Bhagwan

152. The Psychological Society by Martin L . Gross, The Shadow of Dr. Freud, P 233

153. Decline and Fall of the Freudian Empire by Hans J Eysenck, P 149

154. The American Journal of Clinical Nutrition, VOLUME 59, ISSUE5, P1182S-1186S, MAY 1994 by Specker BL,Link : https://ajcn.nutrition.org/article/S0002-9165(23)19590-6/fulltext

155. The cost of reproduction in Female, Modern Biological Theory & Experiment on Celibacy by Jatin Shankar

156. Warning: sex may be hazardous to your health! by Dr Edwin Flatto, New York: Arco, 2nd ed., 1977, Link: https://davidpratt.info/flatto.htm#10

157. The Atharva Veda: Kanda 11 Sukta 7 Mantra 19

158. Shrimad Bhagwat Geeta, Chapter 16 Verse 21

159. Shrimad Bhagwat Geeta, Chapter 3 Verse 43

About the Author

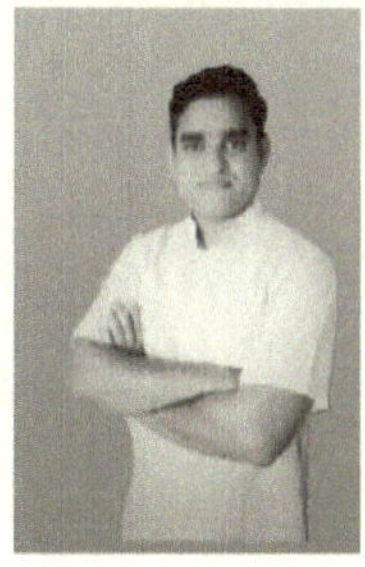

Radheshyam More is a former Naval Soldier, Founder of ManthanHub, PMO recovery specialist, Mindset Coach, Transformation Mentor and author dedicated to helping individuals recover from behavioral addictions and reclaim mental clarity, emotional balance, and inner power. Through his platform Manthanhub, he has guided thousands of individuals through structured PMO Recovery sessions, blending modern neuroscience with ancient principles of awareness, discipline, and energy mastery. His work focuses on sustainable transformation — not temporary control — helping people shift from compulsion to clarity, and from overstimulation to purposeful living.

www.ingramcontent.com/pod-product-compliance
Lightning Source LLC
Chambersburg PA
CBHW031038160726
47991CB00005B/1939